DIAGNOSES
FROM THE
DEAD

The
Book
of
Autopsy

DIAGNOSES
FROM THE
DEAD

The

Book

of

Autopsy

RICHARD A. PRAYSON, MD

EDITOR

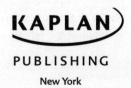

KAPLAN

PUBLISHING

New York

Published by Kaplan Publishing, a division of Kaplan, Inc.
1 Liberty Plaza, 24th Floor
New York, NY 10006

Printed in the United States of America

10 9 8 7 6 5 4 3 2 1

Library of Congress Cataloging-in-Publication Data

Diagnoses from the dead : the book of autopsy / [edited by] Richard A. Prayson.
    p. ; cm.
  Rev. ed. of: Autopsy / Richard A. Prayson. c2007.
  Includes bibliographical references and index.
  ISBN 978-1-60714-082-5 (pbk.)
1. Autopsy. I. Prayson, Richard A. II. Prayson, Richard A. Autopsy.
  [DNLM: 1. Autopsy. QZ 35 D536 2009]
  RA1063.4.P73 2009
  616.07'59—dc22

2009003858

Illustrations by Beth A. Halasz,
Cleveland Clinic Department of Medical Illustrations

The Autopsy

If there were a place where each cared
for his fellow man,
If there were a time when each worked to help
the other,
If that could be, then each death
Would not only be mourned, but studied.
If that could be done, who is to know what
might be?

—WILLIAM H. HARTMANN, M.D. (1985)

CONTENTS

PREFACE

AUTOPSY:
LEARNING FROM THE DEAD

Despite being the focus of considerable controversy since its inception, the autopsy has persisted through the centuries. Unfortunately, this extremely valuable medical procedure may have already reached its zenith. In the 1960s, autopsy rates in teaching hospitals approached 50 percent; since then, rates have declined steadily to less than 10 percent today. This is unfortunate, because autopsies have many uses in addition to determining cause of death. They play a role in establishing public trust in medicine by providing quality assurance for patient care; they offer therapeutic value for grieving family members; and they benefit the population as a whole through detection and surveillance of diseases and environmental hazards. Autopsies are unsurpassed as a teaching aid for medical students, and they afford a unique opportunity to perform certain types of research.

This book is written for people considering careers in forensic science and criminal justice; medical students or professionals in related fields who would like to know more about the practice of autopsy; or anyone who is interested in learning about the subject. We have organized it into 11 chapters focusing on all aspects of autopsy, from the historical perspective to ethical concerns. It covers the purpose behind performing an autopsy, issues surrounding consent, mechanics of how an autopsy is performed, what happens to the body after autopsy, types of information that can be gleaned from an autopsy, special aspects associated with a forensic autopsy, and people's fears and misconceptions regarding autopsy.

This book is unique in that the majority of my coauthors were medical students at the time of its writing. It is my hope that the experience provided these future physicians with an appreciation of the value of the autopsy and how much one can learn—even from those who have completed life's journey.

Richard A. Prayson, M.D.

DIAGNOSES
FROM THE
DEAD

The
Book
of
Autopsy

AUTOPSY 101

After my death I wish you to do an autopsy . . . make a detailed report
to my son. Indicate to him what remedies or mode of life he can
pursue which will prevent his suffering. . . . This is very important,
for my father died . . . with symptoms very much like mine.

—NAPOLÉON BONAPARTE (1769–1821)

NAPOLÉON REPORTEDLY UTTERED these words to his personal physician, Francesco Antommarchi, while in exile on the island of Saint Helena. For years, Napoléon had been experiencing appetite loss, vomiting, bloody stools, and fever. After he died, Antommarchi granted the famous French emperor his final wish, and the autopsy revealed unmistakable signs of stomach cancer.

We actually don't know whether Napoléon's father died of stomach cancer or whether the results of Napoléon's autopsy influenced his son to pursue "remedies" to protect himself from suffering the same fate as his father. Nonetheless, the autopsy unquestionably revealed the cause of Napoléon's death. His request demonstrates that as early as the 1800s, autopsy was becoming accepted as a valuable tool.

This was not always the case. Autopsy has had an uphill climb toward even its current state of lukewarm public acceptance, and it is now experiencing a steep decline in rates of performance.

Fiction fans may love to curl up with a juicy Patricia Cornwell book featuring crime-fighting pathologist Kay Scarpetta, and millions of television viewers are fans of *Bones* and *NCIS*. But mention autopsy outside the context of mystery novels and TV shows, and the only response you're likely to get is an uncomfortable "ugh." Maybe the study of the human body after death is appealing only in fiction.

This shouldn't be surprising. Although the term *autopsy* is familiar, the average person is uninformed about the specific benefits of autopsies. The general public is even less knowledgeable about the actual process of autopsy, from the request to the final report.

These are some facts about autopsy that you probably don't know:

Many previously unknown diseases have been identified through autopsy. With the help of autopsies, a variety of illnesses have been discovered and controlled, including AIDS (acquired immune deficiency syndrome), SARS (severe acute respiratory syndrome), and asbestosis.

Autopsies benefit not only the deceased's family and doctors, they benefit society in general by helping to characterize new diseases and advance the field of medicine.

Contrary to popular belief, doctors are not found negligent in court more often when an autopsy is performed. Studies show that autopsies actually reduce the success of malpractice claims.

Autopsies are an important way to improve the quality of medical care. Autopsies confirm that a correct diagnosis has been made and help to refine medical decisions and procedures. The autopsy can and does contribute to the quality of care in the hospital.

Doctors are not required to perform or observe autopsies during their medical education, which may be one reason for the current low autopsy rate. Some medical schools do not require an autopsy viewing or provide formal education about the process and its benefits.

Such unfamiliarity with the procedure makes some doctors uncomfortable about requesting autopsies.

DEFINING TERMS, FROM A TO P

Autopsy means "an examination of a body after death to determine the cause of death or the character and extent of changes produced by disease." The word comes from the Greek *autopsia,* the act of seeing with one's own eyes.

Necropsy is a direct synonym of autopsy; *nekrosis* in ancient Greek means "deadness," and the suffix *-opsy* refers to study or examination.

You also may hear autopsy called a *postmortem* examination. *Postmortem* means "after death" in Latin.

The definition of *dissect* is to "separate into pieces; expose several parts of for scientific examination." Although dissection clearly is a part of autopsy, it is not the same thing as an autopsy. Dissection may be carried out purely for educational reasons, such as in anatomy courses, without necessarily searching for a cause of death.

The words autopsy and postmortem also carry more general connotations. For example, you might hear about the autopsy of a failed corporate merger or a postmortem discussion after the closing night of a play. Used this way, the terms signify an analysis or evaluation at the end of any process or project.

Such "autopsies" imply that certain questions pertain not only to the end of a project but also to the beginning of the next one: What happened? What was learned? How could this be done better next time?

These questions also apply to autopsy in the medical sense. For example, findings from autopsies often are the cornerstone of hospital morbidity and mortality conferences at which patient deaths are discussed. By discussing what happened in past cases, participants can learn to better care for future patients.

WHODUNIT: PATHOLOGIST, CORONER, OR MEDICAL EXAMINER?

The modern autopsy is performed by a hospital's pathologist, a coroner, or a medical examiner.

A pathologist is a doctor who identifies, interprets, and diagnoses changes caused by disease in tissues and body fluids, either before or after death. A coroner is a public official, sometimes elected and sometimes appointed, whose main duty is to inquire into any death that seems unnatural. In many states, the office of coroner has been replaced by that of medical examiner, usually a licensed pathologist. A medical examiner conducts autopsies on bodies to find the cause of death.

A pathologist needs special training and certification in forensic pathology (the study of pathology as it relates to the application of scientific knowledge to legal problems) to serve as medical examiner and to conduct laboratory or postmortem studies of apparently unnatural or crime-related deaths.

REAL-LIFE CASES

Perhaps the tables are beginning to turn on the public's dislike and distrust of autopsy procedures. Real-life cases have been featured on a number of television shows, including HBO's *Autopsy*, hosted by Michael Baden, M.D., codirector for the Medicolegal Investigation Unit of the New York State Police and formerly New York City's medical examiner for 25 years. *Da Vinci's Inquest* blends real forensic cases with dramatic flair and is shown in more than 45 countries. The reality-based show *The New Detectives* on the Discovery Channel follows forensic scientists as they use their skills to track criminals.

As the appeal of the forensic sciences spills over into real life, the number of applicants to academic programs in forensic science has skyrocketed. It would be a real boon to society if this fascination led to more public acceptance of autopsy.

This little-understood procedure is of inestimable value to public health around the world: it promotes new treatments for diseases, helps prevent threatening epidemics, identifies genetic diseases, and improves the quality of health care. These are just some of the contributions of autopsy in real life.

◆ 2 ◆

SOLVING MEDICAL MYSTERIES

WHAT KINDS OF INFORMATION CAN AN AUTOPSY REVEAL?

A CAR MANUFACTURER wants to improve the safety of seat belts. A medical student wants to learn about the progression of cancer. Family members want to know whether their relative's death was from an inheritable disease. This information and more can be obtained from autopsies.

The three main questions answered through an autopsy are:

1. What was the primary cause of death?
2. The immediate cause of death?
3. The intermediate cause of death?

The *primary cause of death* is the disease or injury that started the events that led directly to death.

The disease, injury, or complication that was a consequence of the primary cause of death is known as the *immediate cause of death*.

The sequence of pathological events leading from the primary cause of death to the immediate cause of death is the *intermediate cause of death.*

For example, a frail, elderly woman in a nursing home falls and breaks her hip. She is in the hospital for a while and develops a pressure wound (bedsore), which becomes infected. The infection becomes systemic (spreads throughout the entire body), and she dies.

The hip fracture was the primary cause of death. Because of the hip fracture, she was bedridden. Being bedridden predisposed her to the development of a pressure wound, which became infected. The infection was the immediate cause of death. The intermediate cause of death was the pressure wound because it linked the hip fracture to the infection.

PITFALLS OF A DEATH CERTIFICATE

Once the cause of death is determined, with or without autopsy, it must be reported properly. A death certificate is a legal document stating the cause of death. It usually has to be filled out within 48 to 72 hours after death by the physician who declared the person dead. The certificate includes:

- The cause of death
- Significant conditions leading to death
- The manner of death (whether it was natural, accident, suicide, homicide, pending investigation, or could not be determined)

This places the responsibility of dictating the primary, immediate, and intermediate causes of death on the attending physician within just days of the death. In the United States, only one primary cause of death can be noted. This can make it hard for a doctor to list the immediate cause of death, when multiple processes appear to have contributed equally. For example, if there's a patient who has had a heart attack and been in a car wreck, how could the physician know whether the heart attack happened before or after the car accident? What should be listed on the death certificate?

Sometimes "cardiopulmonary arrest" is used on the death certificate. This phrase, which is synonymous with death, merely describes the state in which the lungs and heart have stopped working. It says nothing about what *caused* the death. The practice of listing cardiopulmonary arrest on death certificates can lead to the underrepresentation of diseases such as diabetes, dementia, hypertension, infections that are acquired in the hospital, and injury. If one of these is the true underlying cause of death but doesn't get listed, it will be underreported in medical and government statistics.

To further complicate matters, death certificates are often coded by the hospital. The codes are used by the insurance companies for billing and payment, so sometimes the most cost-effective diagnosis is used instead of the most correct.

Another potential problem, when a quick decision about cause of death is demanded, is related to the fact that diseases often are mistaken for one another. The term *mimicry* is used to describe two or more medical conditions that are causally linked but may be mistaken for each other. For instance, take pulmonary embolism (blood clot in blood vessels in the lung) and myocardial infarction (heart attack). If 90 percent of deaths are recorded as myocardial infarction—when in fact 50 percent are from pulmonary emboli—health resources may concentrate on preventing heart attacks when they might well be directed toward preventing and treating pulmonary emboli. In fact, the number of cardiovascular disease–related deaths decreases when autopsy results are used to measure rates.

All this is quite disturbing, since death certificates are used in epidemiological studies as well as to make decisions about public health policy and research funding.

By contrast, an autopsy report allows all the diagnoses to be listed and an accurate disease history to be constructed. (The physician in the above example might know after performing an autopsy on the accident victim which came first: the accident or the heart attack.)

Discrepancies between a death certificate and the autopsy results are important. If the death certificate is amended following an autopsy, many of these complications can be avoided. Unfortunately, this does not happen as often as it should.

HOW THE DEAD HELP THE LIVING

Results from autopsies have determined the effects on humans of environmental and occupational hazards, such as pollution and asbestos. These discoveries were then used to alter adverse conditions, protecting the living from disease and death.

For example, a high incidence of angiosarcoma (malignant tumor) of the liver was discovered from the autopsies of factory workers exposed to vinyl chloride (an organic compound, which is a gas at room temperature; used as an aerosol spray propellant and was once used in hairspray). And autopsies revealed the relationship between long-term asbestos exposure and the development of mesothelioma of the pleura (cancer cells found in the thin layer of tissue that lines the chest cavity as well as the lungs).

In addition, many commonly used products have been improved through autopsy. Cars, seat headrests, and infant and child restraints, as well as protective helmets for biking and motorcycling, have benefited from the use of autopsies of accident victims in evaluating their safety.

Autopsies can link an infectious disease to the cause of death, determining the site of infection and the causative organism (bacterium, fungus, virus, or parasite). In a cancer death, the tumor type, site of the tumor, and the extent of spread, or metastasis, all can be assessed.

Sometimes the approximate amount of time that a disorder was present can also be ascertained. Previous or preexisting diseases can be diagnosed, such as atherosclerotic disease in a patient who dies suddenly of a heart attack.

Certain conditions lend themselves to evaluation by autopsy. Alzheimer's disease, for instance, can be definitively diagnosed only through an autopsy. The doctors may have a clinical suspicion of the diagnosis, which is frequently correct, but confirmation still relies on examination of the brain tissue, which will show the telltale neurofibrillary tangles and neuritic plaques that define the disease.

Of course, an autopsy can simply show gross abnormalities certain to have been the cause of death. Here are some examples of obvious causes of death that can be diagnosed on gross inspection during autopsy:

- Certain cases of heart attack
- Brain hemorrhage
- Ruptured brain aneurysm
- Large pulmonary embolus (clot)
- Rupture of an aortic aneurysm
- Cancer
- Pneumonia
- Ruptured bowel

Just the idea of an autopsy may cause the fainthearted to run away shrieking "Oh, gross!" but in a medical context, *gross* means large enough to be visible to the naked eye. So a gross abnormality does not refer to a condition that grosses out the physician carrying out the autopsy but simply to an abnormality that can be seen with the naked eye.

On the other hand, conclusive abnormalities aren't always grossly evident. The pathologist may need tissue samples to look at with a microscope and a record of events before death to be sure of the cause of death. The following are causes of death that need clarification for certainty (requiring dissection or microscopic evaluation):

- Heart valve problems
- Pulmonary hypertension
- Drug overdose or toxic ingestion
- Narrowing of the veins of the liver
- Cancer type
- Extent of a cancer's spread
- Electrical problems of the heart
- Fat tissue infiltration
- Inflammation (certain types of infection)
- Metabolic diseases

Many times, an autopsy will uncover a previously unknown pathology. The most common pathologies discovered in autopsy are:

- Pulmonary embolism (clot)
- Myocardial infarction (heart attack)
- Tumors (cancer)
- Hemorrhage (bleeding)
- Infection

Pulmonary emboli cause about 200,000 deaths per year in the United States. The embolus is a blood clot that moves through the bloodstream. It can get caught in smaller blood vessels, causing occlusion (blockage). In a pulmonary embolism, a blood clot—which usually develops in the leg (deep leg vein thrombosis)—breaks off, traveling to the lungs, where it blocks blood vessels. If these clots are large enough, they can obstruct large pulmonary arteries, resulting in sudden death. Clinical photographs of a pulmonary embolus, as well as other causes of death discussed below, are present in the book's photographic insert.

A myocardial infarction is an area of dead tissue resulting from an inadequate supply of oxygen-rich blood. In a myocardial infarction, usually one of the main coronary arteries that supply blood to the heart is blocked, causing the muscle tissue to die (necrose). The heart cannot pump blood as well as it should, which can result in death or eventual heart failure.

Tumors are abnormal growths in the body and are also known as neoplasms (literally meaning "new growth"). They can be benign or malignant (cancerous). Benign tumors can grow and put increasing pressure on organs, causing many different problems, including—rarely—eventual death even though the tumor itself is benign. Malignant tumors can spread (metastasize) to distant sites in the body and often cause death. In the United States, common cancer types include lung cancer, breast cancer, colorectal cancer, skin cancer, and prostate cancer.

Lung cancer is the most common cancer type encountered. There is a strong association of smoking with lung cancer. Smoking also causes other pathologies, such as emphysema, which may be evident at autopsy.

A hemorrhage is bleeding into an organ or cavity, usually due to a rupture of the blood vessel. Sometimes, bleeding is not detected until a large amount of blood has accumulated in a body cavity. If enough blood is lost, one can go into shock.

An infection is the result of bacteria, viruses, fungi, or parasitic organisms attacking a part of the body, causing cell death and the release of toxins. A person's immune system is recruited to attack the infectious agent. If the infection overwhelms the ability to fight it off, even with the help of medicine, the person may die. One of the most common fatal infections found at autopsy is pneumonia.

· 3 ·

MORE WAYS
THE DEAD HELP
THE LIVING

AUTOPSIES OFFER THE living a wealth of information that is unattainable by any other means. Although some might argue that computed tomography (CT) scans and magnetic resonance imaging (MRI) studies are cheaper, quicker, and less labor-intensive ways than autopsy to gain information from cadavers, these relatively new methods are not always 100 percent accurate. And even though imaging studies have revolutionized the way that medicine is practiced, they have limitations compared to autopsy.

Such advanced technology can "see" only certain things. For example, imaging studies won't show problems such as very small lesions, metabolic abnormalities, or conditions diagnosed using molecular and genetic tests. Autopsy will.

A big difference between autopsy and CT scans or MRI is autopsy's ability to reliably determine an accurate diagnosis and therefore the real cause of someone's death. About 20 percent of all diseases leading to death are misdiagnosed—a statistic, by the way, that is possible for us to know only because of information from autopsies.

Although we don't like to think about it, it's unlikely that doctors' diagnoses will ever be 100 percent accurate. Why? Well, because of significant advances in medical care today, humans live longer than ever before. This gives us a chance to survive diseases that used to mean certain death. We also develop more complex medical challenges, including the cumulative effects of simultaneous multiple diseases and drug treatments. Despite modern medicine's brilliant new technologies, these factors sometimes make it difficult to determine an exact diagnosis.

Autopsy continues to be the gold standard for pinning down an accurate diagnosis and determining the exact cause of death.

There are many other ways in which autopsies help the living. Let's take a more in-depth look.

HELPING THE FAMILY

When they consent to an autopsy, family members may use the information gained in several ways:

- To help in the grieving process
- To provide assurance that their loved one was diagnosed correctly and received appropriate, quality care
- To discover familial diseases

Here's an example of the positive impact that an autopsy can have on surviving members of a family even though a correct diagnosis wasn't made until the autopsy:

Dawn's father, Mike, had been suffering from several health problems over the past few years. One day he woke up with extremely bad stomach pains that did not get better. His wife, Sara, finally took him to the emergency room, but Mike died later that day.

The doctors told Dawn and Sara that Mike's death was caused by an infected gallbladder. This made no sense to Dawn, since she had heard that doctors could remove a gallbladder fairly easily. Although she did not say so, Dawn wondered whether her mother had contributed to her father's death by hesitating to take him to the hospital. Dawn found herself quite angry at her mother but was unsure how to voice her doubts.

At times, not having a complete understanding of the events surrounding a death places needless stress on surviving family members. An autopsy can help relatives better understand why a loved one passed away. Often, knowing the cause of death is comforting because it can eliminate doubts about the death, as in Dawn's case. It's quite common for surviving relatives to wonder whether there was something they could have done to prevent the tragic event.

Autopsy results demonstrated that Mike didn't die from a gallbladder infection after all. The pathologist who explored Mike's chest and abdomen found a previously undiagnosed metastatic tumor involving his heart. At the very most, Mike might have lived a little longer by coming to the hospital sooner, but he would have likely died from the cancer in short order.

Dawn was somewhat relieved to hear the news. She had hated wondering whether her mother had somehow caused her father's death. The autopsy clearly showed that her mother was not at fault. After the autopsy, this family could continue their grieving process without nagging questions and emotional doubts.

ENSURING QUALITY MEDICAL CARE

Questions often surface surrounding the events that preceded or caused a death, especially if the death was unexpected or unusual.

The family may want an autopsy to ensure that the stated diagnosis was correct and that the treatments given were appropriate. If this was not the case, the family may use autopsy information to decide whether to pursue legal action.

It is estimated that in the United States, about 20 percent of hospitalized patients die each year with missed or incorrect diagnoses. Many of these are inconsequential, but occasionally, significant pathology is uncovered. Performing autopsies more frequently could help uncover these instances as well as improve standards for quality control at health care institutions.

Although we often think of quality control as referring to items like car parts manufactured on an assembly line, medical facilities also need quality-control programs. Autopsies are a source of educational information that helps doctors and hospitals to ensure quality care through refining the way they practice and reaffirming the decisions they make. Ultimately, doctors can use autopsy results to discover their personal areas of inaccuracy and how to do a better job. In fact, hospitals that perform autopsies rely on them for evaluating the accuracy of diagnoses, thereby ensuring the best possible care.

Consider This Scenario

Mrs. Smith, 68, was admitted to the hospital with symptoms of fever, abdominal pain, nausea, and confusion. She told her physician that she was healthy otherwise, but that she had inexplicably lost eight pounds over the past two months. She had dangerously low blood pressure. The concentration of sodium in her blood was abnormally low, and her potassium level was too high. A CT scan of Mrs. Smith's abdomen showed that both her adrenal glands, which sit above the kidneys, were enlarged. Given this clinical information, Mrs. Smith's medical team made a diagnosis of adrenal crisis from Addison's disease.

Addison's disease is a hormonal disorder in which an autoimmune process usually destroys the adrenal glands, which normally make the hormone cortisol. Cortisol is responsible in part for maintaining blood pressure, sodium, and calcium concentrations as well as body weight. All of Mrs. Smith's symptoms seemed to fit this picture of decreased cortisol. An adrenal crisis is a rapid worsening of adrenal gland function, usually the consequence of an unrelated infection. It also is not uncommon for Addison's disease to first manifest—even as adrenal crisis—later in life and especially in women.

Armed with this diagnosis, the medical team proceeded with a treatment appropriate for acute adrenal insufficiency: intravenous fluids and cortisol for the adrenal crisis and antibiotics for any under-lying infection. Mrs. Smith, however, did not improve. The fluids and cortisol could not maintain her blood pressure, and her fever continued despite antibiotics and other fever-reducing medications. She became more disoriented and lethargic, and she died ten days after entering the hospital.

Why had this treatment not worked? Why was Mrs. Smith dead instead of recovering and coping with Addison's disease? Why had she become progressively confused? Both her family and her physicians wanted an autopsy.

Autopsies are fundamental in revealing discrepancies between the diagnosis ascribed to a patient's symptoms and the actual cause of death. Mrs. Smith's autopsy revealed no obvious site of infection. The adrenal glands were increased in size, just as the CT scan had shown. Numerous small blood vessels in both of the glands were filled with large atypical cells, likely the cause of the bilateral adrenal enlargement. In fact, these atypical cells also were found in blood vessels of the lungs, brain, skin, and intestines.

The investigating pathologist stained the cellular contents of vessels from various sites and found one abnormal cell type in each of the samples. The cells showed a cancer: lymphoma. Here was evidence that Mrs. Smith had intravascular lymphoma, a rare, aggressive, and incurable form of cancer in which tumor cells multiply within vessels and clog them.

The Addisonian symptoms observed in Mrs. Smith were related to widespread blood vessel blockage in the adrenals, resulting in the gland's destruction, diminished cortisol production, and symptoms very similar to Addison's disease. Some of Mrs. Smith's other symptoms, such as confusion, can be explained by the brain's being affected by the disease.

Mrs. Smith's family gained peace of mind because they learned the answers to their questions. They weren't interested in pursuing a lawsuit after understanding that this rare type of lymphoma was responsible for the symptoms of Addison's disease.

THE REASONS BEHIND MISSED DIAGNOSES

Why are diagnoses missed until an autopsy is done? Well, for starters, patients typically arrive at a hospital with multiple symptoms. Physicians must take into account all the information and make the best diagnosis they can. When someone has chest pain, for example, a doctor might first suspect a heart attack—although the pain could be due to other conditions such as pulmonary embolism, musculoskeletal problems, or an ulcer. Sometimes, a patient will die before further testing can determine whether the diagnosis is correct. If an autopsy is not performed, an incorrect diagnosis will be listed as the cause of death, with no one the wiser.

Another example is cancer. Usually, the primary site of the tumor is determined so that the disease can be treated appropriately and the risk for relatives estimated. But tumors sometimes originate in different places from those suspected. For example, a patient with lung cancer may present with a seizure, marking a metastasis or spread of a tumor to the brain. Clinically, the doctor might think the patient has a primary brain tumor. Only if a radiographic study of the lung or an autopsy was done would the lung cancer be discovered. So it is possible that what doctors believe is the primary site may actually be a metastatic site, representing the cancer's spread from another site. Radiographic studies are not always useful in sorting this out.

Hemorrhages sometimes cause death if not discovered and treated. Peptic ulcers, gastric erosions, and bleeding of esophageal varices are common causes of hemorrhage. (Varices are dilated veins that can rupture and cause a massive amount of bleeding.) In addition, retroperitoneal (behind the abdomen) hemorrhage is often discovered during autopsy to have contributed to death. Brain hemorrhage is another fatal event that commonly goes undetected until autopsy.

Then there are infections such as pneumonia and rheumatic fever, and infectious agents such as tuberculosis, anthrax, and *E. coli*, which may be uncovered only in an autopsy. Pneumonia, meningitis, infective endocarditis, sepsis, and tuberculosis also are often discovered only postmortem.

IDENTIFYING GENETIC DISEASES

Now that the Human Genome Project has completed its goal of identifying all the approximately 20,000 to 25,000 genes in human DNA, genetics research is revolutionizing the way that doctors practice medicine. It is now possible to probe or test for genetic diseases before symptoms even appear. An increasing number of illnesses have been linked to genetic factors. The possibility to prevent or temper genetic diseases is more real than ever before. How can autopsy help in this exciting arena? Consider the following case:

At 47 years of age, Christine had never been able to give up smoking. She found herself in the intensive care unit of the local hospital with shortness of breath and wheezing. As her symptoms worsened, it became increasingly clear that her lung disease, presumed to be emphysema, was untreatable. She passed away shortly after being admitted. Everyone, including Christine's doctors and family, assumed that her emphysema was attributable strictly to her smoking.

The medical examiner performed an autopsy and was surprised to find that Christine had a diseased liver in addition to her diseased lungs. This finding would not have been consistent with the initial diagnosis of smoking-related emphysema, although the smoking had undoubtedly worsened her condition. Laboratory tests revealed that Christine actually had a rare genetic mutation called alpha-1 antitrypsin deficiency, which contributed to her death. Alpha-1 antitrypsin deficiency is a lack of a protein that blocks the destructive effects of certain enzymes. Without this protein, people may develop emphysema and liver disease.

Christine's case is unusual, as it is rare for a genetic disease to be uncovered during an autopsy. But when it does occur, family members can then be examined or screened for that disease.

In this scenario, it would be important for Christine's children to be tested for alpha-1 antitrypsin deficiency. If they also had the disease, her children, grandchildren, and other immediate relatives could slow the disease's progression through lifestyle changes such as refraining from smoking and not working in dusty environments.

BENEFITS TO MEDICINE AND THE PUBLIC WELFARE

The benefits of autopsy for the medical community and the general public are numerous. Autopsy information helps to:

- Ensure quality control
- Characterize diseases
- Prevent epidemics

- Advance medical education, research, and knowledge
- Raise awareness of health risks
- Develop safer treatments

Let's take a more in-depth look at each of these contributions.

Quality Control

We've looked at quality control from the patient's point of view. Now let's see how autopsy can benefit physicians and other medical professionals in ensuring the highest-quality health care.

Mark, 56 years old, was transferred to the intensive care unit with complex lung and digestive problems. He was put under the care of senior staff member Dr. P. and resident physician Dr. S.

Mark's case was severe, and a diagnosis was difficult, considering the number of symptoms he had. After analyzing Mark's tests, the doctors diagnosed pneumonia, chronic obstructive pulmonary disease, and gastric ulcers.

During the course of the next couple of days, Dr. S. recognized that Mark was not urinating as much as usual and that the area around his stomach felt tense and was painful when touched. He told Dr. P. about his findings, but Dr. P. believed these concerns were relatively minor. He recommended that the young doctor pay more attention to Mark's other symptoms.

The patient's condition worsened, and he died several days later.

An autopsy revealed that Mark had suffered from a severe stomach infection with sepsis (infection in the blood) in addition to the other diagnoses the doctors had made. The infection was causing the decreased urination and the tense and painful stomach.

Because of these autopsy results, Dr. P. changed the way he practiced medicine and improved his care of other patients. Now whenever he sees a patient with decreased urination or a tense abdomen, he makes sure to check for the same kind of infection that killed

Mark. He also informed his colleagues about the situation, and they, in turn, changed their practice methods.

For his part, Dr. S. learned that his findings were of clinical relevance despite his junior status, and he has been reassured about his competence. This will boost his confidence and reaffirm his dedication to details as he advances in his career.

The facts that were disclosed from the autopsy also may stimulate new research that could benefit physicians and patients.

Another way that autopsy contributes to quality control is by giving hospitals reliable statistics for measuring safety and the efficiency of their staff. For example, say that the personnel in a cardiac catheterization laboratory failed to diagnose a specific condition that eventually led to patient death 7 percent of the time. If the average rate of such misdiagnoses in hospitals is less than 1 percent, that means an extra 6 percent of patients treated in this lab are dying unnecessarily. This translates into 60 extra deaths per 1,000 patients per year.

Further investigation would likely uncover a problem in the way the procedure is performed or how patients are taken care of afterward; a solution could then be devised. It would have been thanks to autopsy results that this problem came to light in the first place.

Characterizing a Disease

Characterizing, in this context, means describing a disease's specific qualities. Qualities of numerous diseases and medical conditions have been described more completely after autopsies uncovered clues to their characters.

Atherosclerosis provides a clear demonstration of how autopsies have helped to characterize disease. This condition involves an accumulation of fatty plaques and cholesterols in blood vessels. If the plaques build up and the vessel becomes blocked, a heart attack or stroke may occur.

Some of our most important information on the character of atherosclerosis came from autopsies performed on soldiers who died in combat in the Korean War. As part of the autopsies that sought to characterize trauma, doctors decided to also look at the coronary arteries. They were amazed to find that more than 77 percent of the soldiers autopsied had cholesterol plaques lining the walls of their arteries. Why was this surprising? Prior to these autopsies, atherosclerosis was thought to develop only after a long life of eating foods high in cholesterol. The unexpected cholesterol accumulation in the arteries of these men—mostly in their twenties—showed that atherosclerotic buildup starts much earlier than thought, maybe even in childhood.

This valuable information changed the way that heart disease was treated and researched. For example, it has led to the development of age-appropriate screening exams to help prevent heart disease.

Some Diseases Discovered and Characterized by Autopsy*

Heart
- Tricuspid valve insufficiency due to a metastasizing tumor
- Atheromatous embolism
- Asymmetric cardiac hypertrophy
- Dissecting aneurysm
- Cardiomyopathy
- Subaortic muscular stenosis
- Rheumatoid disease of aorta and aortic valve
- Complications of cardiac surgery
- Diseases of the conducting system
- Hypertrophic subaortic stenosis
- Mitral valve prolapse

[*] Modified from R. B. Hill, R. E. Anderson, "The Recent History of the Autopsy," *Archives of Pathology and Laboratory Medicine,* vol. 120 (8) (August 1996): 702–712.

Lungs
- Diffuse alveolar damage
- Shock lung
- Respiratory distress syndrome
- Oxygen toxicity
- Pneumocystis pneumonia
- Infantile respiratory distress syndrome
- Legionnaires' disease
- Pulmonary alveolar proteinosis
- Desquamative pneumonia
- Lipid pneumonia
- Diffuse interstitial fibrosis

Liver
- Viral hepatitis
- Alpha-1-antitrypsin disease and cirrhosis
- Jamaican bush tea disease
- Infantile kernicterus
- Neonatal giant cell hepatitis and biliary atresia
- Vinyl chloride and angiosarcoma of the liver
- Tumors and hyperplasia due to oral contraceptives
- Aflatoxin-induced liver disease and tumor

Kidney
- Damage due to use of diethylene glycol as drug vehicle
- Renal effect of potassium deficiency
- Elucidation of various types of glomerulonephritis
- Necrotizing papillitis and interstitial nephritis due to phenacetin abuse
- Renal development malformation in polycystic diseases
- Renal vein thrombosis syndrome
- Scleroderma kidney

- Acute tubular necrosis (ATN) injury
- Atheromatous embolic renal disease

Blood, Bone, and Spleen
- Role of spleen in thrombocytopenia purpura; value of splenectomy
- Secondary hemochromatosis
- Syndrome of myeloid metaplasia
- Effects of incompatible blood transfusion
- Aplastic anemia, granulocytopenia, thrombocytopenia as a complication of drug therapy

Gastrointestinal
- Whipple's disease
- Protein-losing enteropathy
- Congenital intestinal atresia
- Pancreatic cystic fibrosis
- Vascular insufficiency syndrome and hemorrhagic enteropathy
- Protein and potassium loss from villous adenoma

Endocrine
- Complications of diabetes mellitus in vessels, eye, nerves, kidneys
- Aldosteronism (Conn's syndrome)
- Hypercortisolism
- Multiglandular endocrine syndromes, Zollinger-Ellison syndrome

Nervous System
- Spongiform encephalopathy (Creutzfeldt-Jakob disease)
- Progressive multifocal leukoencephalopathy

- Adrenoleukodystrophy
- Subacute sclerosing panencephalitis
- Carotid artery insufficiency and thrombosis
- Dementia with Lewy bodies
- Alzheimer's disease

Other
- Toxic shock syndrome (TSS)
- *Ebola* virus
- AIDS
- Lyme disease

Preventing Epidemics

Autopsies help doctors and scientists to recognize and combat emerging diseases, protecting the general public as they do so. No matter how rapidly technology advances, new diseases continue to originate. One recent example was the SARS outbreak, which first appeared in Asia in 2003 and caused a scare all around the world. Until then, the scientific community had known little about the disease in terms of its mechanism, detection, and treatment. Being able to conduct autopsies allowed physicians and scientists to quickly understand more about it, as well as to develop tests for the SARS virus.

Advancing Medical Knowledge

Suppose that a 55-year-old man, in excellent physical shape and with no known health problems, swerves in front of a car on his daily bicycle ride and is killed. A cursory exam might suggest that his death be attributed to the massive trauma from the accident, and this may be correct.

However, it also may be discovered during an autopsy that the bicyclist had severe carotid artery atherosclerosis (blockage in a neck artery) that had never been symptomatic. His atherosclerosis had caused a minor stroke when his heart rate increased from bicycling. This caused him to become dizzy, which was why he swerved into the path of the car.

Undetected atherosclerosis in the carotid artery is fairly common. Information gained at autopsy helped the development of screening tests for carotid artery disease. Such screening procedures, administered early in life, may find disease sooner, thereby allowing for early intervention.

Now imagine that you are the child of the bicyclist mentioned above. Twenty-five years after you made the decision to allow your father's autopsy, you were screened and treated under new guidelines established in part due to your father's unfortunate demise. The value of autopsy begins to take on new meaning.

Autopsy also yields new connections and observations that advance scientific knowledge. One observational study of autopsied patients showed that approximately 27 percent were afflicted with a condition known as patent foramen ovale. In patients with this condition, a flap connects the two upper chambers (atria) of the heart. Everyone is born with this flap, which allows the fetus to get oxygen-rich blood from the mother without breathing, but normally it closes after birth. Because of this discovery, research into patent foramen ovale was pursued over the past 25 years, and a connection was made between patent foramen ovale and stroke and migraine headaches. Work during the past decade has led to an experimental treatment for both stroke and migraine, in which a surgeon closes this defect in the heart. Whether or not this treatment turns out to be effective, the research and innovation leading to its invention likely never would have existed without the original autopsy.

Raising Awareness

Autopsies have shown that certain diseases often aren't diagnosed because they don't cause symptoms. A good example is prostate cancer. Knowing that this cancer is often asymptomatic until it is advanced has led to a far greater emphasis on men getting regular screening tests for early detection. Early detection leads to early treatment, saving lives.

Autopsy data also are useful for studying the patterns of a disease: how it is spread, its risk factors and predisposing features, and which groups are at higher than usual risk. Thanks to patterns discovered by autopsy, people can protect themselves from health problems because of a better understanding of:

- The variability of certain diseases in different populations (for example, a higher incidence of high blood pressure in African-Americans)
- Whether they are at increased risk
- How the disease is—and isn't—transmitted

The scientific community and government funding agencies use patterns to decide which diseases should have higher priority in funding for research and what directions that research should take.

Safer Treatments

Many of today's standard treatments were developed or perfected from knowledge gained from autopsies. For example, pathologists performing autopsies discovered that chest tubes, which are designed to be inserted in the chest to help patients breathe more easily, were sometimes accidentally being inserted into patients' livers instead. With this autopsy-derived information, the chest-tube technique was modified, and now the problem is rare.

Autopsies have been tremendously helpful in expanding physicians' understanding of immunocompromised patients—those who are unable to fight typical infections from which a healthy person recovers more easily. Autopsies on immunocompromised patients showed that fungal, not bacterial, infections were interfering with their quality of life and eventually leading to death. Since doctors had been treating these patients with antibiotics, which are ineffective in fighting fungal infections, a new therapy was clearly required. Immunocompromised patients suspected of infection are now treated with antifungal medications as well, and there has been a huge decrease in the number of deaths from fungal infection.

Autopsy has also helped physicians evaluate the effectiveness or toxicity of therapies. Autopsies of cancer patients, for example, linked the chemotherapeutic drug doxorubicin to heart failure. The discovery resulted in an adjustment in the drug's dosage to minimize the possibility of heart failure while maximizing its cancer-killing potential.

Every year, new prosthetic devices are created to assist human bodies to function better and longer. An autopsy can show the effect over time of such devices. In the 1960s, the prosthetic heart valve, which can be sewn in place to help people with faulty valves, was at the cutting edge of available technology. Postmortem results helped developers perfect the valve's size, shape, and materials even more. Autopsy results also helped physicians determine who could safely receive such a device and who couldn't.

Other medical devices and procedures have been improved, including indwelling feeding tubes, endotracheal tubes for airway management and mechanical ventilation, and performance of cardiopulmonary resuscitation.

· 4 ·

HISTORY OF THE AUTOPSY

AUTOPSY AS A method of exploring and discovering the cause of death did not come into practice until the 18th century. It grew out of the practice of dissection and the study of anatomy.

As far as we know, the ancients did not perform autopsy. Even the Egyptians, famously concerned with embalming their dead kings, did not carry out autopsies. It's true that organs were removed, dried out, and treated with a carbonate salt to prevent decay, but they were not studied or examined in any way.

The main purpose of mummification was to protect the body's beauty and preserve it so that the dead person's spirit had a place to dwell during the afterlife. Following Tutankhamen's death in circa 1323–1325 B.C., 15 mini-coffins containing his embalmed organs were in his tomb, ready to accompany him to the afterlife.

Even though *autopsy* and *necropsy* both stem from ancient Greek words, the Greeks didn't dissect human cadavers. As in many cultures, they believed that after death, the human spirit could not participate in an afterlife if the body had been altered or mutilated.

EARLY FIGURES IN AUTOPSY

Ptolemy I of Egypt (367/366–283 BC) was probably the first ruler to allow the dissection of cadavers, mostly executed criminals. Not only did he give the royal okay to these procedures, it is said that he participated in some of them.

One of Ptolemy's goals as a ruler was to make his capital, Alexandria, a great center of science and medicine. Because of this, he allowed anatomists Herophilus and Erasistratus to dissect and study corpses.

Herophilus, who lived around 335–280 B.C., performed numerous public dissections of human and animal cadavers. He is believed to be the first physician to dissect human beings and has been honored with the title father of anatomy. Among other findings, Herophilus discovered the anatomical distinction between arteries and veins, as well as the existence of and difference between motor and sensory nerves. This revolutionized surgery during his lifetime and afterward.

Herophilus also catalogued many body parts that still lacked names. The confluence of sinuses—a point at the back of the brain where some of its veins join together—is known still as the torcular Herophili.

Just after Herophilus made his mark as the father of anatomy, Erasistratus began making a name as the father of physiology. (Physiology is the study of the normal functions of the body.) Around 250 B.C., Erasistratus left his birthplace, Ceos, for Alexandria, which was flourishing with anatomical study and research. There he made many contributions to the understanding of the human body. Although he incorrectly described the circulation of the blood, Erasistratus accurately noted that the heart prevented backflow of the blood and that the epiglottis covered the windpipe during swallowing. Like Herophilus, his work was done primarily on criminals who had met with the death sentence.

The writings of Galen, formally Claudius of Pergamum (circa A.D. 131–201), forged many more connections between anatomy and physiology. Galen was born in what is now modern-day Turkey and settled in imperial Rome as a surgeon for injured gladiators as well as the personal physician of the emperors Marcus Aurelius, his son Commodus, and later Septimius Severus.

On the Usefulness of the Parts of the Body is Galen's masterwork, containing a set of meticulous descriptions of his anatomical and physiological findings. For centuries after his death, Galen was regarded as the preeminent authority on human anatomy and physiology. This, and the prominence of the book, is actually quite strange, since it appears that Galen drew all his conclusions from animal studies; he did not dissect human cadavers. Despite this major shortcoming, Galen deserves mention in any history of autopsy because he is credited with the idea that postmortem symptoms of illness and disease are mirrored in the "affected part of the deceased," an idea that paved the way for modern-day uses of the autopsy. Galen's mistakes were not discovered for 14 centuries, even though the study of human anatomy continued in some cultures.

Frederick II, the 13th-century Holy Roman emperor and German king who had a strong interest in science, decreed that medical schools must receive at least two bodies of executed criminals each year for study and demonstration. (It seems that crime didn't pay in the 13th century any more than it did in Ptolemy's time.)

As the Renaissance began, anatomy teachers and students in medical schools did not perform dissection themselves. Rather, they would sit in an operating theater in which a cadaver was opened by a third party, a lay dissector. This dissector, known as a "surgeon," was often a wage laborer or a prisoner. He was paid very little or nothing at all to make physical contact with human remains, then considered a demeaning act. Professor and students participated only in the intellectual aspects of medicine, which remained separate from the experiential.

Anatomy professor Andreas Vesalius (1514–1564) changed the paradigm of separating intellectual and experiential work. As an undergraduate at the University of Paris, Vesalius was apparently so taken with courses in dissection and anatomy that he would often go to Paris's deteriorating cemeteries late at night to study the bones of skeletons. This extracurricular activity seems to have paid off. Immediately following his graduation, Vesalius was appointed lecturer and anatomical prosector (a person who prepares a dissection for demonstration) at the University of Padua in its department of surgery.

Recognizing that animal study was an inferior and inexact route to human anatomy, Vesalius used human cadavers. He also saw that medical training influenced dissection ability and that he could reveal and describe human anatomy better than could a laborer or prisoner.

Any controversy that surrounded this young professor's personal dissections of human cadavers must have been silenced with the publication of his seminal work, *De Humani Corporis Fabrica Libri Septem* (*The Seven Books on the Structure of the Human Body*), in 1543. Vesalius was only 28 years old when this work, known today as the *Fabrica*, was first published. These volumes were and remain accurate documentation of human anatomy and made it clear that Galen's theories were incorrect. In addition, the *Fabrica* contains numerous depictions of abnormal anatomy, an early cataloguing of pathological processes.

After the publication of the *Fabrica*, medical schools began to require that their students dissect human cadavers. This acceptance of dissection, as well as reports of pathological findings, reinforced the nascent field of forensics: the use of science and technology to investigate and establish facts in criminal or civil courts of law. (For more information on forensics, see chapter 6.)

In the wake of the *Fabrica*, the autopsy came to be an essential element of medical, educational, and legal investigation. Vesalius's alma mater the University of Padua endured as the European seat of anatomy. From this institution came the most influential successor to Vesalius, Giovanni Battista Morgagni (1682–1771), who chaired the anatomy department for 56 years.

Morgagni expanded the understanding of pathology. His 1761 work, *De Sedibus et Causis Morborum per Anatomen Indagatis* (*On the Seats and Causes of Diseases Investigated by Anatomy*), catalogues more than 600 complete dissections involving disease processes and associated anatomical changes. *De Sedibus* demonstrated the causal relationship between physical findings at death and manifestations of disease during life. Pathology, the study of the essential nature of diseases and the structural and functional changes produced by them, had become a unique discipline.

Examination of the human body consequently became more of an exact science, and physicians, students, and other practitioners of autopsy reaped the benefits of having standards with which to compare their findings.

During the 19th century, centers of academic medicine throughout Europe and the United States founded pathology departments. Autopsies investigating hospital deaths continued to be performed by clinicians. No pathologist was arguably more versed in the autopsy during this period than one particular Austrian who proved its merits: Karl Rokitansky (1804–1878).

Rokitansky personally performed more than 30,000 autopsies during his 45-year career at the Vienna General Hospital. Such a singular focus gave him the experience necessary to relate pathological findings to the manifestations of disease that his patients had experienced. It also allowed him to catalogue pathological findings in more detail than ever before.

For example, Rokitansky discovered that acute endocarditis, an often fatal inflammation of the lining of the heart, can be caused by bacteria. He had seen, on simple inspection, bacterial colonies in the heart of a patient who had succumbed to endocarditis. He also classified types of pneumonia based on the region(s) of the lung that each type affected. Such discoveries proved the power of simple gross pathological examination and the necessity of autopsy in revealing and describing human disease.

Autopsies became increasingly common in the 19th century. Not only were they used in hospitals, but they also were becoming a mainstay of criminal investigations. One case involved a young slave suspected of being pregnant and having been poisoned. Her planta-tion owner ordered an autopsy to prove himself innocent of both the impregnation and poisoning. Dr. J. O. Sharber, a private physician, performed the autopsy and published his findings in the *Nashville Journal of Medicine and Surgery* in 1853:

> "[The autopsy] resulted in revealing the true cause of the patient's death, which was not in consequence of having received a poisonous draught, but caused by internal hemor-rhage. In laying open the abdomen, it was found to be filled with coagulated blood and serum. This hemorrhage had originated from an ulcer on the right margin of the fundus [body] of the uterus. . . . I regard the ulcer as being one of carcinomatous character, and as having been of several years standing. The cervix and os uteri [opening to the fundus] are very obnoxious to cancerous affections; but I do not know that I ever knew the fundus uteri to be the seat of carcinoma before this instance."

The woman was neither pregnant nor poisoned. She had long-standing uterine cancer, which had eventually caused her to bleed to death. The plantation owner was exonerated.

Cases like this one demonstrate that during this era, autopsy and pathology were becoming widely understood and accepted disciplines by physicians and lay people alike (although even Dr. Sharber declared himself as having a personal "aversion . . . to such inspections").

However, autopsy was not without its drawbacks. A student of Rokitansky's, Ignaz Semmelweis (1818–1865), observed that the deaths of new mothers from childbed fever at the Vienna General Hospital seemed to be associated with the fact that delivering physicians routinely arrived straight from the morgue after performing autopsies. Without knowledge of a microbial basis for infectious disease, hospital workers did not routinely wash their hands between tasks or patients, as they do now. Semmelweis was ridiculed for suggesting a link between the autopsies and the deaths, and he died before the significance of his observation was recognized.

Nonetheless, the 19th century ushered in more advances in medical science and practice than did any previous historical era. Surgical principles and techniques were refined to minimize blood loss and to reduce death rates from operative procedures. New anesthetic agents came into common use, minimizing surgical pain and other pain. Microbes were discovered as the agents of infection, and infection-control guidelines greatly and dramatically reduced deaths.

Despite these rapid medical advances, diagnoses were often inaccurate, and the medical community did not understand the reasons behind many diseases.

The autopsy continued to develop and improve during this time. It was especially helped by the development of histology: the examination of tissues at the cellular level (such as sperm and blood cells) and organisms such as parasites. Histology transformed the performance of autopsies and greatly increased the amount and type of information that could be gleaned from a cadaver.

Simultaneously, improvements in the microscope also had a favorable impact on the autopsy. Designed in its early stages by Anton van Leeuwenhoek (1632–1723), the microscope was quite a sophisticated piece of equipment 200 years later. Its reliability and widespread use produced an explosion of information in many different sciences, including medicine.

A noteworthy proponent of microscopic study for pathology and the autopsy was Rudolph Virchow (1821–1902), one of the first cellular pathologists to use histological examination along with gross (or macroscopic) examination of organs and tissues during autopsy. Using this approach, Virchow characterized a case of leukemia, a cancer of the blood cells. Leukemia is one of many diseases that does not give many outward clues about its cause or mechanism of development.

Virchow's publication on the anatomy and histology of the leukemia case was one of the earliest formal reports of this cancer. His cellular work helped to show that the macroscopic autopsy, performed so frequently by Rokitansky, was often limited in its ability to describe diseases completely. Virchow was so well known that one of the two main methods of autopsy procedure was named for him and carries his name today.

THE MODERN AUTOPSY

Today, an autopsy has many fancy submacroscopic tools at its disposal: more specific histological stains (sometimes involving antibody binding and called immunohistochemistry), molecular characterization techniques (looking for proteins and other markers), and genetic testing (looking at DNA). Pathology's next frontier is to continue to relate molecular and genetic information to established knowledge of gross anatomy and histology.

Even in this era of technology, however, many times just a peek inside a body with the naked eye is enough to give a conclusive answer about the cause of death. The fundamental tasks of the autopsy are as important as ever: macroscopic observation of the exterior of the body and of the internal organs, followed by appropriate tissue samplings and histological preparations.

Autopsy's current form stems from its historical roots of natural curiosity about the human body, anatomical and physiological investigation in the academic setting, and the formal establishment of the field of pathology to characterize disease symptoms and signs in light of abnormal anatomy.

Plummeting Autopsy Rates

Hospital-based cadaveric studies in the 19th century, those by Karl Rokitansky in particular, represent the heyday of the autopsy as the cornerstone of pathology. Such reliance on the procedure continued into the 20th century.

However, rates of investigation of hospital deaths by autopsy have plummeted over the past few decades. In the 1950s, autopsies were performed on close to half of all hospital deaths in the United States. Now that number has dropped to about 6 percent.

In chapter 11, we'll explore the possible reasons for this decline. For now, let's continue to deepen our understanding of autopsy and take a look at how an autopsy is conducted.

· 5 ·

HOW IS AN AUTOPSY DONE?

AN AUTOPSY IS a complex procedure with many steps and stages, but there is no difficulty in understanding the basic techniques and what may or may not be learned from them. Of course, numerous differences in procedure may occur, depending on the practitioner and institution where the autopsy is being performed.

WHO CONDUCTS THE AUTOPSY?

In most cases, the person performing the autopsy is a medical doctor who has specialized training in pathology. Pathology is the scientific study of the nature of disease and its causes, processes, development, and consequences. Pathologists have the skills to diagnose diseases and obtain information from the gross and microscopic appearances of tissue in the living as well as in the dead.

Others who might perform the autopsy or parts of it include the deceased's physician, a mortician in the funeral home, or the *diener,* an individual who specializes in the evisceration portion of the autopsy procedure, which is performed only at the next of kin's request. The evisceration portion involves actually removing the organs from the body. Removing and examining an organ sometimes can reveal more information than examining it in place.

Because certain religions have specific rules about how a body is handled after death, a religious representative may attend the autopsy to ensure that the guidelines are followed. (See more about religion and autopsy in chapter 9.) In addition, partial autopsies may be requested, where limited prespecified portions of the normal autopsy are performed. Partial autopsies are carried out according to the wishes of the next of kin. For example, a family may not want the brain removed and examined for fear of leaving the deceased's face mutilated (although this does not happen). Or the next of kin are reluctant to allow a complete autopsy but believe it is important to know just what happened to the person's heart. In this case, only the heart would be removed and examined.

WHAT IS THE ROOM LIKE?

The location of the autopsy room can vary greatly; however, it is common for the room to be near the morgue, where the bodies of deceased individuals are stored prior to transportation or autopsy. If the place of the procedure is not near the morgue, cold storage near the autopsy room is required. (The book's photographic insert includes photographs of the autopsy room, as well as other tools used during an autopsy.)

The actual room where the autopsy is performed is pretty much the same, whether it's in a county morgue, a hospital setting, or a private mortuary. Any differences between rooms is based on the number of procedures performed, whether observers regularly attend, the economics of the facility as a whole, and performer preferences.

An important functional characteristic of room design is that it needs to be easily cleaned. Sloping floors, specially designed work tables, and sterilizing facilities are essential. Ventilation is designed to prevent the return of air to other hospital or work areas, and to turn over the air in the autopsy room in a relatively short period. These factors all reduce the possibility of infection by waterborne and airborne diseases. There may be additional precautions taken by having a showering and dressing area available to personnel and observers.

Special design qualities that are fairly common include cold storage or refrigeration for excised specimens, dictation equipment to allow the performer to make oral notes, a separate station for dissecting organs, a vacuum machine to clear fluid from the body, and a photography station to take pictures of various findings.

AT THE START

The autopsy begins when the body arrives from the morgue with the deceased's medical records, proper identification, and a valid, completed consent form. (For more on consent, see chapter 8.) It's important to have documentation linking the body to its proper identity. Most commonly, this is either a toe tag or wristband.

At this point, the physician reviews the medical records, looking for any previous medical conditions or procedures as well as other pertinent information that could help in framing the autopsy. If a medical record is not available, the pathologist may contact the personal physician or caregiver. All this information helps give direction to the autopsy and raises questions that need to be answered.

The pathologist does several things before even picking up a scalpel. He or she must take "universal precautions" against communicable or infectious diseases before having any contact with the body, even when the risk of infection appears low. Although there is no worry about transmitting infection to the (dead) body, it's possible for the pathologist and assistants to contract diseases from the deceased.

Each person involved in the autopsy therefore dons a surgical gown, face mask, safety glasses (similar to those used by a construction worker), two pairs of latex or nitrile gloves, and shoe covers. Additionally, the pathologist will usually change into scrubs (the blue or green cotton clothing commonly worn by hospital staff) to prevent contaminating his or her street clothes. The doctor also ensures that there is adequate ventilation and that all devices—such as the suction hose, drainage system, and bone saw—are clean and in good operating condition.

These precautions guard against diseases known to be infectious and transmissible at autopsy. Two examples are tuberculosis (TB) and the more obscure Creutzfeldt-Jakob (prion) disease. TB particularly affects the lungs and was very common prior to the antibiotic era. The combined use of antibiotics and quarantine procedures has largely limited this type of bacterial infection, but certain antibiotic-resistant strains still exist and may be spread very easily. The mycobacterium organisms that cause TB can live for days, even weeks, within the lungs of a deceased individual. The organism is easily aerosolized when infected tissue is exposed or cut. Without protective measures, this would put the pathologist at obvious risk, particularly from a lung resection. (Tissues removed at autopsy can be placed into formalin for fixation prior to processing. The formalin also serves to kill viable TB organisms that may still be alive in the tissue.)

Creutzfeldt-Jakob disease, or the related bovine spongiform encephalopathy, which is acquired from consuming contaminated beef from a cow with mad cow disease, can also potentially be transmitted at autopsy. This infection is transferred through an "infectious" protein (prion protein) that has certain characteristics. This prion protein can damage brain tissue. Unfortunately, infection with prions is a uniformly fatal condition.

The diagnosis is frequently made postmortem during autopsy. The prions can be transmitted through an open wound or by contact with mucous membranes.

EXTERNAL EXAMINATION

Now the autopsy itself can begin. The body is weighed and measured lengthwise. If it's a forensic autopsy, the body may be X-rayed at this stage to help determine the location of an assailant's bullet or suspected areas of trauma. (For more on forensic autopsy, see chapter 6.) Evidence of child abuse, such as multiple recent and healed fractures, may be detected on X-rays.

Photography may also be used at this time to obtain pictorial evidence of wounds. Unusual bodily characteristics such as a cleft palate, an abnormal chest configuration, or spinal column abnormalities such as scoliosis may be photographed.

Microbiological cultures to test for bacteria or fungal organisms causing infection would be taken at this point in the autopsy. These cultures can glean information related to infectious organisms that may have contributed to the death. Samples of blood, hair, skin, or the eyes' vitreous fluid may be obtained. These may be helpful in toxicological evaluation (looking for evidence of drug or alcohol use or poisoning).

The pathologist then performs a careful visual inspection of the entire body, taking note of any abnormalities and measuring dimensional oddities. All orifices, including the ears, nose, mouth, anus, vagina, and urethral opening, are inspected. The mouth and teeth are inspected as well as the tissue covering the inside of the oral cavity. The neck is inspected for any bumps and swellings, and the trachea (windpipe) is palpated and manipulated to examine the thyroid gland.

The skin color and quality over the entire body are examined to look for signs of diseases that can manifest on the skin. For instance, yellow skin (jaundice) is a telltale sign of liver dysfunction. The locations and designs of tattoos, scars, and needle tracks are recorded. This is most important in cases where the body has not been readily identified—a situation that happens less often in the clinical setting. Tattoos and scars are unique markers of individuals and are of particular interest to the forensic pathologist and criminal investigator.

In the case of a person who died in the hospital, the pathologist then carefully documents any procedures the deceased has undergone, noting evidence of intravenous or arterial blood lines, catheters, pacemakers, chest tubes, and so on.

In patients who have had recent surgery, the pathologist will document the appearance of any surgical site, noting its location, how intact it looks, and whether it seems infected. The abdomen and genitals are examined, along with any other areas that seem abnormal either from the medical records or by visual exam. For instance, the pathologist might examine the pelvic region of the deceased more closely if an untreated hip fracture was noted in the patient's history.

INTERNAL EXAMINATION

The internal examination begins with what is called the Y incision. A riser of some sort (wood block, rolled towel) is placed underneath the shoulder blades to raise the upper portion of the chest (thorax). A scalpel is then used to make an incision from the front of one shoulder (acromial process) to the front of the other shoulder, arching down to below the center of the rib cage.

From the center of this flattened U-shaped incision, a vertical incision is made all the way down the front of the body to the bottom of the pelvis (pubic symphysis). It is important to note that this incision avoids the belly button (umbilicus) and does not penetrate bone or cartilage, just muscle and fat.

The thickness of the abdominal fat may be measured before the belly (abdominal cavity) or the thorax is entered. How thick the abdominal fat is can indicate whether the person was at risk for several diseases, including common ailments such as heart failure and diabetes. Scissors, instead of a scalpel, are used to cut through the abdominal wall, to avoid cutting too deeply and damaging an organ.

Once the abdomen is opened along the vertical line, the flaps that have been made are flipped back, allowing one to view the inside of the body. Each of the three flaps of skin, muscle, and fat must be reflected back (pulled out of the way) while being freed from their body attachments. This is especially important along the sternum, where the pectoralis muscle origins are located; the chest muscles meet in the middle of the breast plate. The breast muscles and glands (mammary glands in women) will be examined with their own incisions (if warranted), in a search for any potential malignancies or masses. If a suspicious lesion is found, the pathologist may take samples to be viewed later.

The internal abdominal cavity is examined even before organ removal. Inspections of the linings of the abdominal cavity and all the membranes that support and connect the cavity walls to the organs are viewed and examined. The internal fat layer that droops down over the stomach and small intestines (omentum) is inspected. The relative positioning or relationship of organs to one another is noted to rule out certain developmental abnormalities that result in uncharacteristic positioning of the organs.

The pathologist looks for evidence of fluid collection (ascites) or blood collection (hemorrhage) in the abdominal cavity. The ribs are examined to see whether there are any fractures—for example, due to chest compression during cardiopulmonary resuscitation. If a urine sample is required, a needle is inserted into the bladder before removal of the organ.

The abdominal organs are then removed, including the liver, pancreas, large and small intestines, and spleen. These may be removed either while still attached to one another (en bloc) or piecemeal.

After the abdominal organs have been taken out, it is time to remove the chest plate (sternum) to access the heart and lungs. The ribs are connected to the chest plate by cartilage. Additionally, the collarbone (clavicle) connects to the top of the chest plate, and this joint must be removed. Usually, rib cutters are used for this job, cutting each rib up to the collarbone on both sides of the body about halfway to the arm (midclavicular line), as shown in the smaller, semicircular cutting line (see photographic insert). A bone saw may be used to free the collarbone from the chest plate, at the sternoclavicular joint connecting the two. This joint is very rigid, and movement is not normally noticed in everyday life. Once the chest plate is freed by cutting along the aforementioned lines, the whole plate is lifted off, leaving an additional cavity. This is known as the thoracic cavity, the inside of the chest where the heart and lungs are located.

With the anterior (toward the front) portion of the chest wall removed, the thoracic cavity is now open, providing an excellent view of the lungs and heart. Many diseases can show up in these areas.

After the sac around the heart is removed, the position of the heart and its size are noted. Enlargement of the heart (hypertrophy) or certain parts of it is a common finding in some diseases, such as long-standing hypertension (high blood pressure). The lungs are inspected closely, noting any lesions or whether the lungs are collapsed (pneumothorax). The color and quality of the lungs are important because these factors can provide clues as to the health and social habits of the deceased. The lungs may look black (black lung), resulting from years of work in a coal mine. Another possibility is that the lungs have many slimy black deposits along the inner membranes (these can be seen externally without dissection), suggesting that the deceased was a smoker. Even people who live in a city have blacker lungs than someone who has lived in the country, away from pollution.

In addition to examining the lungs and the heart (noting their positions and quality), any fluids in the cavity are sampled, and their location and amount are noted. The thymus gland, a component of the immune system, also would be examined at this point.

REMOVING THE ORGANS

There are several techniques for organ removal and many variations in each, depending on who is performing the dissection and the specific goals of the procedure. Two basic approaches can be taken: the *Virchow method* and the modified *von Zenker method*. The Virchow method involves removing each organ one by one and dissecting it separately. Many forensic pathologists use this method. (See chapter 4 for more information on Virchow and his distinguished career.)

The von Zenker method (named for Friedrich Albert von Zenker, a German physician and pathologist who lived from 1825 to 1898) calls for removing the entire organ block at one time, then dissecting specific organ systems. Many pathologists prefer this method, as it may reveal certain pathologies the Virchow method may not.

Whichever procedure the pathologist uses, the goal is the same: to examine the organs and the body cavity linings for any abnormalities. This is important for finding diseases or injuries that have created tissue abnormalities beneath an organ's surface. If there are other clues evident from the autopsy or the medical records, the pathologist may allot extra time or special techniques to studying a selected organ or organ system. Key areas for study frequently include the heart, lungs, genitals, pancreas, kidneys, liver, and intestines.

Each organ is carefully dissected. Solid organs, such as the liver, may be cut into thin sections (*bread-loaf cutting*). Each cut surface is examined carefully. These large slices make it much easier to view the organ's internal components to identify congenital defects, cancer, cystic disease, cirrhosis, or necrosis (tissue death).

EXAMINING THE ORGANS

Dissecting an organ makes storing and handling it easier, especially if it needs to be studied at different locations or requires multiple tests from different labs. It also allows the pathologist to see certain lesions that might not be discernible if only the outside of the organ were examined.

Examining the excised heart can yield a great deal of information about a person's health and fitness. The pathologist notes any surgical abnormalities, such as coronary artery bypasses or valve replacements. Birth defects also would be noted.

The layer of fat surrounding the heart is measured as is the size of certain muscular sections, such as the left ventricular myocardium. The organ size and weight are recorded.

Hollow organs, such as the intestines, are cut open so that their inner linings can be examined and the contents analyzed. Someone who has committed suicide by overdosing on pills may have partially digested pills still in the stomach.

TISSUE SAMPLING

Tissue from each organ and lesion may then be taken (called *sampling*) and prepared so that it can be looked at under a microscope. Sometimes the only way that a physician can get a true understanding of a disease's process is by microscopic examination.

The tissue is prepared by slicing extremely small, thin segments—usually no more than a half inch to one inch in width and length—from the organ. The segments are embedded in paraffin wax; this forms a *tissue block*.

This block can be mounted in a machine known as a *microtome*, which can slice off even thinner tissue sections (only 4 to 5 microns thick; thinner than a strand of hair). These tissue sections are placed on a glass slide, stained, and examined using a microscope.

The blocks and slides can last for many years, and it is common for hospitals and other institutions to store them for long periods. The rest of the organs are usually discarded or can be returned to the body if requested.

REMOVING THE SKULL AND
THE BRAIN

The brain and spinal cord are very important parts of an autopsy. In some cases, examining the brain postmortem is the only way to make an accurate, definitive diagnosis of disease.

The technique of brain removal is frequently misunderstood, causing significant anxiety for family members. What is most important to understand is that the deceased is able to have an open-casket viewing, with his or her appearance unaltered to the casual observer. The pathologist uses precise techniques so as not to change the facial features or the shape of the skull.

To begin removing the brain, the pathologist uses a scalpel to cut the scalp from just behind one ear, over the top of the head, to just behind the other ear. The front skin flap is then pulled down over the face and the rear flap back down to the neck. This exposes the skull without making an incision that would be visible during a funeral.

With the scalp displaced and the skull exposed, the top portion of the skull can be removed, exposing the brain. Skull removal used to be performed using a *bone chisel,* notching through the hard bone of the skull above the ears completely around the head. It is much more common now to use a power tool known as a *bone saw.* This type of saw uses a vibrating motion to make a clear cut around the skullcap, easing its detachment. After this cut is made, the skullcap that is removed is about the size of what would fit underneath a baseball cap. (See photo insert.) Careful attention to the removal process allows the skull to be placed back on the deceased after the brain is removed. The skin is replaced for funeral preparation.

Within the skull is the brain, covered by a tough sheath called the dura. The brain now can be removed with its coverings attached. However, the contour of the bone on the inner aspect of the skull and its brain attachments are complex; removing the brain without damaging it may be difficult.

The brain is first freed from its main posterior (situated from behind) attachment, then pulled backward so that the anterior portion of the skull is visible. Here the olfactory bulb (nerves responsible for detecting odors), the optic nerves (nerves responsible for seeing), the vasculature (blood vessels going to and from the brain), and the spinal cord can be severed. The brain is now completely free from its attachments and can be taken out for dissection and examination.

REMOVING THE SPINAL CORD

The spinal cord is removed next. This is a highly labor-intensive process and is usually approached in one of two ways. The first is an anterior approach, meaning from the front. This involves removing the vertebrae from within the abdominal and chest cavities, even as high as the middle cervical (neck) vertebrae.

This is accomplished by cutting through the high disc in the neck and a lower disc in the small of the back and removing this entire segment of vertebrae. This leaves the spinal cord exposed from the small of the back to the middle of the neck. (See photo insert.)

The cord now can be excised by (1) cutting the dura away from its attachments, taking care not to cut into the spinal cord itself; (2) transecting the lower nerves near the small of the back (cauda equina); and (3) lifting the whole cord up and toward the head while severing the spinal nerves.

The second approach to removing the cord is from the posterior, or back side. Although this may take even more time and effort than removing the cord from the front, it usually enables a more thorough examination while preserving the integrity of the spinal cord to a greater degree.

For this approach, the body is placed facedown on the table. The skin and musculature of the back are displaced with a midline incision; all soft tissue covering the spine from the rear is dissected and pulled laterally (sideways) to display the posterior aspect of the spinal column. Now the bone saw can be used to cut through the posterior portion of the vertebral arch. Care always is taken here not to cut so deeply as to damage the spinal cord itself. With the cord visible, the dura can be freed from its attachments and the cord removed from the body as mentioned above.

STUDYING THE BONE MARROW

The last area of study is the bone marrow. Bone marrow is important in the production of blood and immune cells, and some may be sampled during an autopsy, especially if there is reason to believe that a disease of the marrow, such as leukemia, existed prior to death.

As its name suggests, bone marrow is found within the bones of the body. The flat bones, such as the pelvis, contain red marrow, and the long bones, such as the femur (thigh bone), contain yellow marrow. Common sampling locations include the ribs and the pelvis.

Smears can be made for examination in the pathology laboratory. This type of preparation involves taking a small amount of tissue and literally smearing it onto a glass slide. It is then stained so that it can be looked at under the microscope.

COMPLETING THE AUTOPSY

There may be other procedures done at this point, depending on the findings so far, the medical history of the deceased, and any limitations placed on the autopsy by the next of kin.

The eyes may be examined for abnormalities and signs of certain diseases, such as diabetes, glaucoma, melanoma, or infection. The veins in the legs may be opened and examined to see whether a large venous thrombosis (blood clot) is present. Breast tissue may also be removed and sent to the pathology laboratory to check for breast cancer.

When organ and tissue removal are complete, the abdominal and thoracic cavities are sewn closed, and the body is cleaned and released to the funeral home. All contaminated materials are either disposed of in proper biohazard bags or *autoclaved* to decontaminate and kill potentially infectious agents. Autoclaving is heating under pressure, in this case to disinfect or sterilize.

THE AUTOPSY REPORT

During the autopsy procedure, a large amount of physical evidence is generated, both in written form and in prepared tissue. This is directed to the appropriate parties for their review. Institutions differ somewhat in the exact ways that they report autopsy findings, but certain basic characteristics of reporting are necessary for accuracy and efficiency. These include the *autopsy face sheet* and the *clinical-pathological summary*.

The autopsy face sheet includes the most basic and fundamental pieces of information that identify the deceased and provide an overview of the findings:

- The name of the deceased, Social Security number, and patient number
- Where the autopsy was performed
- A case number (as a way for the pathology department to identify the procedure and correlate it with stored tissue samples and other information)
- The patient's age and race or ethnicity
- Date and time of death
- Whether the autopsy included forensic procedures
- The party who granted permission
- The autopsy date
- Name of the pathologist performing the autopsy

Other items that might be included are:

- The deceased's address and occupation
- Pending studies
- The name of the physician of the deceased

The most basic diagnostic information is also presented on the face sheet. This includes the actual cause of death. Normally there is a brief history of the illness, with the findings listed so as to show the progression of the disease to the moment of death. Alternatively, the information may be listed in order of importance or relative to each organ system involved in the diseased state.

The clinical-pathological summary is more in-depth, incorporating detailed information from the clinical scenario, the details of the gross autopsy results, and any other studies—including microscopic findings. The pathologist uses all the data and the autopsy findings to produce an objective time frame and a judgment on the cause of death and the disease process that led to it.

Gross anatomical findings are a key part of this record, as are the results of the tissue studies. All this information, in combination with the medical records, helps to generate the hypothesis about the cause of death or confirm/refute the findings of the physician who pronounced the individual dead.

Information pertaining to the process of the disease is provided, and the clinical-pathological summary may correlate premortem signs and symptoms with the anatomical and microscopic findings.

RETAINING MATERIALS

How autopsy documents and physical specimens are kept is an important part of the autopsy. Accurate paper and tissue records, which may benefit future patients, should be retained so that the rights and wishes of the deceased are honored and maintained.

Different materials are held onto for varying lengths of time. On average, the authorization forms and records are kept for at least a year, while the quality-assurance documents are saved for twice that long. Wet tissue may be kept for as long as 6 months, usually preserved in formalin, while paraffin blocks are usually held for a minimum of 5 years. Microscope slides (*histological sections*) and the autopsy report normally are kept for a minimum of 20 years; however, this may be extended if there is ample storage space.

While the regulations for how long each of the above should be kept vary from state to state and institution to institution, it is universally required that the documents and tissue be kept confidential to respect the deceased and any loved ones affected by the information.

· 6 ·

FORENSIC AUTOPSY

MODERN FORENSICS IS the use of science and technology to investigate and establish facts in criminal or civil courts of law. Forensic autopsies capture our imagination. From *Quincy M.E.*, the TV series of the 1970s and 1980s in which actor Jack Klugman found clues on bodies, to the newer *CSI: Miami*, or sensational real-life murder trials like O. J. Simpson's, there has been a fascination with the forensic autopsy and its ability to unravel the cause of death in even the most mysterious of circumstances.

Let's start with the basics: what *is* a forensic autopsy? A forensic autopsy is performed when a medical-legal issue has been raised about the death of an individual. The goal of the forensic autopsy is to determine the cause of death and how the death came about. The person's death is often sudden, unexpected, unexplained, or otherwise suspicious. Such cases also include those with significant injuries, drug abuse, or suspected drug toxicity; those who die while in police custody; and anyone who doesn't have a physician to sign a death certificate—for instance, someone who hasn't seen a doctor in years.

Of course, the autopsy is not the only tool used to discover how someone died. An investigation often involves the work of law enforcement officials and may also entail interviews with physicians, analysis of the person's medical history, and interviews with family, friends, acquaintances, and/or other witnesses. If foul play is determined, the evidence found at autopsy may be used in a court of law.

FROM JULIUS CAESAR UNTIL TODAY

The forensic sciences—the study of evidence discovered at a crime scene and used in a court of law—date back to antiquity, but autopsy, which is a part of the forensic sciences but by no means the entire field, did not come on the scene until later. Until the 12th century, decisions about how someone died were based primarily on investigation of the circumstances surrounding the death. Little attention was paid to the body itself, and dissection was generally not performed.

There are some known exceptions. A physician in Rome is reported to have examined the body of Julius Caesar after he was assassinated and determined that only one stab wound in the chest caused his death. The other 22 wounds on his body were not felt to have been contributing factors.

In the year 1250, a Chinese handbook titled *Hsi Yuan Lu* (translated variously as *The Washing Away of Wrongs* and *A Collection of Vindicated Cases*) provided guidelines for examining bodies after death. In addition to detailed descriptions of various wounds caused by blunt versus sharp objects, the author explained how to tell whether an individual found in the water had died of drowning or had been killed before being left in the water. Similarly, this text described how to determine whether a burned individual had died before sustaining the burn injuries.

As early as 1302, in the Italian city of Bologna, an unidentified local magistrate asked that the body of a victim be examined to determine whether any criminal activity had killed him. Although the autopsy did not reveal a guilty party, the case was nevertheless a milestone because of its recognition that a body might betray its cause of death.

Later, a physician from Florence, Antonio Benivieni (1440–1502), is said to have examined 15 corpses as part of criminal investigations and helped to attribute guilt through his findings.

It was not until the publication of Vesalius's *Fabrica* about a half century later, though, that findings from autopsy could truly be corroborated with the normal and abnormal anatomy documented in the textbook.

The development of forensic pathology dates to the early 1500s, with the publication of the Bamberg Code. This code underscored the significance of forensic pathology by allowing medical testimony to be an integral part of trials or decisions about the manner of death in infanticides, homicides, abortions, and poisonings.

By the latter half of the 16th century, official medicolegal autopsies were being performed, and shortly thereafter, formal lectures on the subject of forensic pathology were being held at Germany's University of Leipzig.

WHO CONDUCTS THE FORENSIC AUTOPSY?

Oddly enough, doctors were left out of the autopsy business until 1860, when the Code of Public General Laws in the state of Maryland required that the coroner or his jury had to have a physician in attendance in cases of violent death. The choice of physician was left to the discretion of the coroner, but soon thereafter it was mandated that the governor appoint a physician as the sole coroner.

In 1877 in Boston, Massachusetts, a statewide system was adopted requiring the coroner to be replaced by a physician who would be referred to as a "medical examiner." The jurisdiction of the medical examiner was confined to those persons whose deaths were related to violence.

Over the next several decades, the role of the coroner's or medical examiner's office widened to include investigation of all deaths related to criminal violence, casualties, or suicide; sudden deaths in individuals who were apparently healthy or who had not been attended by a physician; and deaths of prisoners. The coroner or medical examiner was also responsible for investigating any suspicious or unusual deaths.

The first statewide medical examiner system was not established until 1939 in Maryland. This allowed for investigation of a broad spectrum of cases and gave the medical examiners authority to order an autopsy when deemed appropriate. The medical examiner was appointed by a group consisting of professors of pathology, an executive officer of the state and the city health department, and a superintendent of the state police. This effectively removed the medical examiner's appointment from the list of political appointments and set the stage for the development of career forensic pathologists.

THE CORONER SYSTEM

The U.S. coroner's system has its roots in a system initially developed in England during the Middle Ages. In 1194 three knights and one clerk were elected in each county to be "keepers of the pleas of the crown." These crown representatives, or "crowners"—later corrupted to *coroners*—were expected to collect funds such as taxes and forfeit fees derived from criminal activities and death. In addition to the crown representatives, there were justices, similar to traveling judges, who could request that coroners perform various administrative or other duties within the region where they were appointed.

Certain responsibilities soon became associated specifically with the coroners, including holding inquests over dead bodies, the inspection of an individual's wounds, recording accusations against individuals, and arresting accused individuals in suspected homicides.

Coroners were also authorized to gather witnesses or suspects and appraise and safeguard the land or goods that might later be forfeited by reason of the guilt of the accused individuals. Eventually, the coroner's job became focused solely on investigation.

The English coroner's system was transported across the Atlantic by the colonists. One of the earliest recorded descriptions of the duties of the coroner in America dates to 1640.

Autopsy examination of bodies was recorded as early as 1647 in Massachusetts as part of the teaching of medical students. Shortly thereafter, in 1665, a forensic autopsy was recorded in Maryland when one Mr. Francis Carpenter was accused of murdering his servant, Samuell Yeoungman. The coroner's report absolved Mr. Carpenter of any blame.

Today, forensic autopsies can be performed by medical doctors with different specialties, but many states and local governments hire a forensic pathologist. (A forensic pathologist has special training in analyzing and interpreting injuries and drug toxicity, and in determining what factors have a role in causing death.) These individuals are referred to as medical examiners.

Not all counties in a given state use the medical examiner system, however. Some use coroners. In this system, the coroner is an elected official who may or may not be a pathologist or even a physician. In many instances, the coroner is a qualified pathologist, but not always.

Whether a coroner or medical examiner system is used often boils down to an issue of manpower in a given location. The number of trained forensic pathologists is relatively low, and there may not be enough to cover certain rural areas. In general, the incidence of

CHAPTER 6

violent crimes in underpopulated, rural areas is relatively low, which
makes justifying a full-time forensic pathologist difficult.

The function of the coroner, in contrast to the medical examiner,
is to declare an individual deceased, identify the body, notify the next
of kin, collect and return any personal belongings on the body to the
family, and sign the death certificate.

In cases in which nonphysician coroners think that an autopsy
should be performed, they may seek out the services of a medical
examiner.

LOOKING FOR ANSWERS

When a forensic autopsy is performed, there are often three key
pieces of information being sought:

1. The cause of death
2. The mechanism of death
3. The manner of death

The forensic pathologist must be familiar with a variety of findings. Gunshot wounds, sharp trauma versus blunt-force trauma,
drug overdoses, asphyxia, drownings, hangings, strangulation, child
abuse, sudden infant death syndrome, sexual battery, and electrocu-
tion are among the many pathologies that may be uncovered in a
forensic autopsy.

The cause of death, from the perspective of forensic autopsy, is
defined as the disease or injury responsible for the sequence of events
that leads up to a person's death.

The cause of death can be divided into:

* The *proximate cause of death*
* The *immediate cause of death*

The proximate cause of death is the event that initiates the continuous, linked sequence of events that results in death. These events must not have been interrupted by any other significant, independent, intervening event (such as the victim of an auto accident dying from cocaine abuse while recovering from his or her injuries).

The immediate cause of death is defined as the complication or sequence of events of the underlying cause of death. For example, a person who has been severely beaten and robbed is found in a park. At the emergency room, he is found to have several broken bones, which are repaired surgically. The surgery appears to have been successful; however, while in the hospital, the patient comes down with pneumonia and dies.

In this scenario, the underlying or proximate cause of death would be the beating, which required hospitalization and surgical intervention. The more immediate cause of death is the pneumonia, which the victim would not have developed had he not been hospitalized due to the beating.

The *mechanism of death* refers to alterations in the person's physiology or biochemistry that underlie the death. Examples of mechanisms of death include congestive heart failure related to fluid overload of the heart, arrhythmia (irregular heartbeat), sepsis (widespread infection), renal (kidney) failure, and asphyxia.

On death certificates, the term *cardiorespiratory arrest or cardiopulmonary arrest* is often listed as the cause of death. But this really isn't the cause of death. Rather, it is a description of the *state* of being dead—that is, when the heart and lungs stop working.

The *manner of death* attempts to explain how the cause of death arose and is generally categorized as either natural or violent.

Natural deaths are caused entirely by normal aging or an underlying disease, such as coronary artery disease, diabetes, or asthma.

If any injury is involved in the death, the manner of death is classified as violent. *Violent deaths* may be subcategorized as *accidental* (not intentional), *homicide* (deliberately or inadvertently inflicted by another individual), *suicide* (injury that is self-inflicted), or *undetermined*.

If the manner of death is designated as undetermined, but evidence turns up later elucidating more clearly what happened before death, the manner of death may be changed.

Particular *causes* of death can have different *manners* of death, depending on how an injury is sustained. For example, a gunshot wound in the head can be a homicide, a suicide, or an accident.

The following four sample cases present the corresponding causes, mechanisms, and manners of death for each situation. This is precisely the information that a forensic pathologist would try to uncover.

The Unfortunate Case of the Shop Owner

A 52-year-old shop owner was closing up late on a Friday afternoon. Two youths entered the store carrying guns and demanded that he give them the money in his cash register. The shop owner refused and reached under the counter for a gun he kept hidden. One youth shot the man twice in the stomach. Both youths fled.

The shop owner managed to drag himself to the telephone and call 9-1-1. The ambulance arrived quickly and rushed him to the hospital. He was taken immediately to surgery, where it was noted that one of the bullets had perforated his colon in two places. The bullets were removed successfully.

During the next few days, the man appeared to be recovering well from his surgery. On the night before he was supposed to be discharged, he developed a fever. The doctors did a routine evaluation, including microbiological cultures of his blood. The blood cultures showed bacterial organisms similar to those usually found in the colon.

The shop owner developed abdominal pain and was found to have an infection of the abdominal cavity, or peritonitis. Despite antibiotic therapy, he died of overwhelming infection 11 days after the initial gunshot injury.

The cause of death was the gunshot wound, which started a lethal and unbroken sequence of events for the shop owner. The more immediate cause of death was the infection he sustained from the perforation of his bowel and the peritonitis.

The mechanism of death was infection. Even though the man died a week after the gunshot wound, his death was not directly due to being shot.

Still, the manner of death would be ruled violent and homicide. This is because the gunshot wound started a series of events that resulted in the man's death.

The Case of the Late-Night Jogger

A 48-year-old woman was jogging alone in a park at night when a masked man jumped out from behind a bush and grabbed her. She screamed and attempted to kick her assailant. She didn't realize that he was holding a gun, which discharged. The bullet lodged in her back. The assailant ran.

Fortunately, she was found ten minutes later by a pair of joggers who called the police. At the hospital, the victim was found to have a bullet lodged in her thoracic (midback) vertebrae, which caused a fracture of the vertebrae and a paralyzing spinal cord injury.

When she was finally discharged from the hospital, she had to live in a nursing home, since she was unable to take care of herself. Periodically, she would develop decubitus ulcers (also known as pressure wounds or bedsores) on her buttocks. The sores developed because she couldn't change positions in bed. Fifteen years after the gunshot wound, she died from septicemia related to infected decubitus ulcers.

Her cause of death, despite the lapsed period of time, was the gunshot wound. Because of it, she was paralyzed and therefore prone to developing decubitus ulcers, which eventually caused the septicemia that ultimately led to her death.

The mechanism of death was related to the infection and septicemia, similar to the first case.

The manner of this death also would be categorized as violent and homicide.

The Case of the Hot-Dog Calamity

A six-year-old boy was enjoying a summer day at a park near where he lived with his parents and two older brothers. The brothers had finished swimming in the lake and were ready to enjoy a traditional summer picnic dinner of hot dogs, hamburgers, corn on the cob, and potato salad.

The boy told his family that he needed to use the bathroom and walked off in the direction of the toilet, hot dog in hand. His mother shouted after him to make sure he finished the hot dog before he used the facility.

After about 15 minutes, his mother became concerned that he had not returned and walked toward the Port-a-Potty. She found him on the ground, unconscious and not breathing. The boy was rushed to the hospital but was found dead on arrival with a chunk of hot dog blocking his airway.

The cause of death was aspiration, from choking on a hot dog.

The hot dog blocked his airway, resulting in death by asphyxia, which was the mechanism of death.

The manner of death would be ruled violent but accidental.

The Case of the Depressed Executive

A 29-year-old executive had recently gone through a divorce and had lost custody of her two children to her ex-husband. She had been seeing a psychiatrist for depression and was having trouble sleeping. She was taking medications for both conditions.

She was feeling particularly depressed after her boss put her on probation, explaining that her work was not up to par and that she was forgetting important details, which had resulted in critical mistakes.

The woman decided she that couldn't go on anymore. She wrote a note to her mother saying that life had become impossible to bear and everyone would be much better off without her. Two days later, concerned that she had not shown up for work or called, her boss called her home and then called the police. She was found dead at home by the police. Both bottles of her medication were found next to her bed, emptied, along with a spilled glass of gin. There was no evidence of foul play.

Toxicology levels showed fatal levels of medication and a moderately high level of alcohol in the woman's blood.

The cause of death in this case was the overdose of medication combined with alcohol.

The mechanism of death was likely related to respiratory failure secondary to the medication.

The manner of death was ruled violent and a suicide.

FORENSIC AUTOPSIES VERSUS HOSPITAL AUTOPSIES

Some factors distinguish a forensic autopsy from an ordinary, hospital-based, nonforensic autopsy. The hospital autopsy attempts to associate the patient's medical history and findings with the findings at autopsy, while the forensic autopsy usually tries to make correlations with the terminal events or scene of death.

The hospital autopsy is more focused on disease, whereas forensic autopsies often focus on trauma-related injury and drug toxicity (although they also evaluate natural deaths). While the hospital autopsy is focused on the mechanism of death, the forensic autopsy is looking for the cause and manner of death as well as the mechanism. The hospital autopsy is subject to strict medical confidentiality guidelines; forensic autopsies are generally a matter of public interest and record.

A hospital-based autopsy requires legal permission from the next of kin; forensic autopsies do not. They can be performed by legal authorization or mandate. Families certainly have the right to voice an objection to a forensic autopsy, but ultimately the decision lies with the coroner or medical examiner.

Determining Details of a Death

Although the forensic autopsy may follow the same procedure as the hospital-based autopsy, it can deviate in a number of ways. In some instances, the medical examiner or coroner will visit the death scene, either prior to or following the removal of the body. The visit may provide useful clues and information. For example, the body's position may show whether the person died there or had been moved and put in that position after death.

Bodies of the dead are often placed in bags in order to protect evidence that could be lost during transport. Sometimes the body is wrapped in a clean sheet to help preserve evidence and prevent contamination before it is brought to the morgue.

The medical examiner or coroner will conduct a careful external examination of the dead person's clothing. Before the clothes are removed, photographs may be taken for documentation. In criminal cases or when foul play is suspected, clothing and valuables are inventoried, recorded, secured, and then turned over to the police or to the laboratory for analysis.

Once the clothing is off, the medical examiner will look carefully at the outside of the body. Nail or hair samples, semen, gunshot residue, fibers of various sorts, paint chips, or other objects can potentially provide useful clues as to what happened. In a homicide investigation, the hands of the deceased often will be placed in paper bags at the scene to preserve such kinds of evidence.

The medical examiner may use ultraviolet light to locate secretions on clothes or skin. These secretions—semen, blood, saliva, urine, vaginal secretions, and sweat—tend to fluoresce.

X-rays may be used to locate bullets. Fingerprints are often taken and may yield a positive identification. Frequently the pathologist will draw a body diagram and document on it anything discovered during the external examination.

Photographs of injuries are taken either by the medical examiner or someone else working in the medical examiner's office. If there is excessive blood or gore, usually it is cleaned prior to photography so that it won't be considered inflammatory or prejudicial and therefore dismissed in court.

All tissue specimens, body fluid specimens, and foreign objects, such as bullets collected during the autopsy, need to be treated as potential evidence in a future criminal or civil trial and must be handled very carefully. The *chain of custody* must be respected so that the whereabouts of the potential evidence are known at all times and the materials cannot be tampered with by outside parties. Each item must therefore be appropriately labeled, including items that will be turned over to others for either transport to a laboratory or analysis—for example, bullets to a ballistics lab.

To make certain there are no mix-ups of specimens or samples, they are treated much like registered letters. All persons handling or transporting a specimen must sign a piece of paper attached to it, indicating their purpose, as well as the date and time of receipt.

Toxicology, which is the study of drugs, medications, and poisons (including their sources, chemical composition, action, tests, and antidotes), is an important part of forensic practice. Specimens are generally obtained for toxicological analysis whenever any of these substances is suspected.

Jane and John Doe

In contrast to the hospital-based autopsy, the deceased in a forensic autopsy may need to be identified. Identifying a body may be challenging at times, particularly with bodies that have been exposed to the elements or are partially decomposed. *Forensic entomology* uses knowledge about insects in various stages of development to help determine the approximate time of death when a body has been left outside. Since many insects have well-established life cycles, it is possible to make some general conclusions about how long the body has been outside, based on the stage of insects infesting the body.

Dental records, if available, provide a unique profile of the individual and can be used for identification. The pathologist would compare *antemortem* (before death) dental X-rays with ones taken of the dead person's mouth. In 1775, Paul Revere was able to identify a general, Joseph Warren, by his dentures after the Battle of Bunker Hill. Revere had made the dentures and recognized them, even though the general's body had been buried in a mass grave.

Skeletal evaluation also can provide general information about height, gender, race, and general age to try to identify a John or Jane Doe.

Sudden—and Perfectly Natural—Death

Although we commonly associate violent deaths with forensic autopsy, most cases investigated in a medical examiner's office are sudden and unexpected natural deaths. One type or manner of death may mimic another, and family members and law enforcement officials may want to establish not only the natural disease that caused the death but also that no injuries played a factor. This is particularly true when the events surrounding the death happen so quickly that it is impossible to establish the cause or manner of death with sufficient certainty to relieve suspicions of foul play or to illuminate violence as a factor.

In fact, in many cases, death by natural causes may resemble death related to violent causes. For example, a person might be found apparently drowned, the victim of an attacker. At autopsy, it could be discovered that the person suffered a ruptured cerebral aneurysm (burst blood vessel in the brain) that caused immediate death and the subsequent drowning.

Or a death may look like a homicide or suicide but later be found accidental. Take the case of a driver found dead behind the steering wheel of his automobile after it ran into a tree. The autopsy showed numerous external and internal injuries of the chest and abdomen, including multiple fractures and laceration of the heart, lungs, and liver. Toxicology levels showed no drugs or alcohol. There was no significant internal bleeding. But examination of the heart and arteries showed severe atherosclerotic disease of the coronary arteries and evidence of myocardial infarct (heart attack).

The man's death was attributed to heart disease, not the car accident. A heart attack presumably caused the car accident and all the other injuries. Sorting out the cause of death with coexistent pathologies can be challenging.

Making the distinction is critically important. If a natural death is characterized as a homicide, for example, the police could be obligated to search for a nonexistent murderer (among other troubling possibilities). Labeling someone's death a suicide may have significant ramifications on life insurance policies or burial rights, not to mention the emotions of surviving family and friends.

Sometimes, the cause of death may be established beyond any doubt. In other cases, it may be established by a history that can be confirmed or supported by findings at autopsy. Unlike on TV, the cause of death can't always be determined with complete certainty. But the forensic autopsy certainly gives it the best shot—er, takes a good stab at it—um, you get the idea.

The causes of sudden and unexplained natural death in this country are quite numerous. In the United States, the most common reasons include cardiovascular disease, including atherosclerotic heart disease, myocardial infarction, valvular heart disease, hemorrhage, or bleeding in the case of a ruptured vessel resulting from an aneurysm or dissection, where layers of the blood vessel wall divide by blood.

Other sources of bleeding may include intracerebral (brain) hemorrhages, ulcer disease of the stomach, or esophageal varices (dilated vessels that are prone to rupture; they usually develop in patients with liver disease commonly associated with alcohol use).

The occlusion, or blockage, of vessels by thromboemboli (blood clots), particularly in the involved lung (pulmonary embolism), can cause sudden death.

Other potential causes of natural death include infection, seizures, and asthma, to name just a few. While many of these entities are the focus of attention in the hospital-based autopsy, they may be merely a portion of the pathology that a forensic pathologist encounters in any given case.

· 7 ·

WHAT HAPPENS TO THE BODY AFTER AUTOPSY?

IN MYSTERY STORIES, the murderer often has trouble disposing of the corpse. Fortunately, in polite society, there are rules about what happens to a dead body, including after it is autopsied.

In general, the most common method employed in disposition of the body involves embalming followed by a funeral service and burial; in recent years, cremation has also gained increased acceptance. The decision about these matters is usually made by the next of kin in conjunction with a funeral director, unless the deceased person made his or her wishes known beforehand. These parties also decide about the preparation of the body, the specific type of coffin or casket to be used, and the body's final resting place, which may be in a grave at a cemetery, in an aboveground mausoleum, or in what is called a columbarium: a wall of niches specifically created to hold urns with ashes of loved ones who have been cremated. Columbaria may be located indoors or out.

Autopsy would not affect any of these decisions. After the autopsy, the coroner, medical examiner, or hospital notifies the funeral home so that transportation of the body to the funeral home can be arranged.

EMBALMING, FROM THE 19TH CENTURY TO NOW

Modern embalming, a procedure used to disinfect and preserve dead human bodies, originated in the 1860s. Before the Civil War, Dr. Thomas Holmes (1817–1900) developed an embalming fluid that he then used to prepare the bodies of dead soldiers for their transport home to their families. Dr. Holmes apparently moved from battlefield to battlefield, setting up makeshift embalming stations and using a rubber squeeze ball to pump the fluid into the deceased. Reportedly, he embalmed more than 4,000 bodies in this fashion.

Today, embalming fluid is injected into arteries using a motorized injector pump. If an autopsy has been performed and the arterial system has been disrupted, the embalming fluid can still be injected using a hypodermic needle.

Organs removed from the body are soaked in embalming fluid. An autopsy compound may also be applied prior to returning them to the body. These are absorbent powders or gel desiccants that are used to preserve, disinfect, and harden body organs or other remains that are in an advanced state of decomposition—as might happen if a body has been exposed to the elements or isn't found for several weeks after death.

More Facts about Embalming

The U.S. Department of Health and Family Services has published standards for embalming. Regulations require that embalmers hold a funeral director's license or an apprentice funeral director's certificate.

The embalming itself may be performed in a certified funeral establishment, hospital, facilities approved by the local medical examiner or coroner in the event of a disaster, accredited mortuary schools or medical schools, and in private homes under specific circumstances.

There is no particular delay between the autopsy of a body and its embalming. It is embalmed as soon as it has been transported from the autopsy site to the funeral home.

There are a variety of reasons for embalming:

- **Public health and sanitation.** The fluids used for embalming have disinfectant properties.
- **Travel time.** Embalming the body allows people who need to travel considerable distances to attend the funeral an opportunity to do so.
- **Additional time to mourn.** Embalming also affords families and friends additional time with the body of the deceased as part of the grieving process.

The embalming fluid is colored pink to give the body some color. Following the embalming process, the mortician makes the body presentable for public viewing. Cosmetic preparation of the body, or *restorative art*, as it has come to be known, uses various waxes and makeup to restore head and facial features to normalcy, if necessary. A properly performed autopsy should not interfere with the corpse's looks, however. (For more on how an autopsy is carried out, see chapter 5.) The process of restorative art is said to help mourners confront the reality of loss while trying to minimize the negative effects of disease, suffering, death, and decomposition.

While the funeral industry clearly supports the practice of embalming, and many view it as a necessity, it is not required by law. The next of kin may choose to have no embalming or partial embalming, in which only a part of the body is treated.

CREMATION AS AN ALTERNATIVE

The funeral home can also handle arrangements for cremation.

In preparing a body for cremation, any metal such as dental fillings or devices such as pacemakers must be removed. Then the body is placed in a cremator, which, under very intense heat, reduces it to ashes. The temperature ranges from 1,400 to 1,800 degrees Fahrenheit.

It usually takes two to two and a half hours to reduce the body to ashes, which fall into a container that can be removed. Cremations are done individually to ensure that the deceased's identity is maintained and that people's remains are not mixed together. If bone fragments remain, they are processed into small particles and placed into a container with the ashes.

All Christian denominations allow cremation; Orthodox Judaism and Islam forbid it. (For more on religion and autopsy, see chapter 9.)

Many states require that cremations be authorized by the coroner or medical examiner, since the ability to determine the cause of death is obviously compromised by the process. Certain states have specific minimum time limits before a cremation can occur; bodies are usually refrigerated or may be embalmed during this time, depending on the time interval and plans for public viewing.

Following cremation, the deceased's ashes may be buried, retained by someone (usually in an urn), scattered (with permission of local authorities if in a public place), or placed in a columbarium.

MAKING ARRANGEMENTS
AFTER A DEATH

A number of decisions concerning the disposition of the body need to be made in consultation with the funeral director. In many cases, the first issue to be considered is embalming, followed by burial or cremation. Details to be addressed include preparation of the body, the date and time of the service, the type of service that will be performed, the type of coffin that will be used, the location of the final resting place for the remains, transportation to and from the funeral, the death and/or funeral notices for the newspaper, and arrangements for the wake.

Certain documents will be required:

- Death certificate (Every death needs to be officially recorded. A physician usually provides a medical certificate indicating the cause of death. Based on this document and other information, a death certificate is then issued. The estate generally cannot be administered without a death certificate.)
- Social Security card
- Marriage certificate
- Birth certificate
- Veteran's papers, if applicable
- Deceased's will, if there is one
- Life insurance policies, if any

The deceased's employer should be notified, allowing coworkers to find out about funeral arrangements. This also allows the employer to officially end the person's employment, which often has implications for pension funds, compensation, and medical insurance. Notification of organizations that the deceased belonged to may facilitate informing friends of the death and may provide the family a certain amount of support.

FUNERAL DIRECTORS AND AUTOPSY

One of the factors cited as contributing to declining autopsy rates is the attitude of funeral directors. There are no obvious incentives for funeral directors to participate in the autopsy process, and there are several potential disincentives.

Funeral directors have influence in two ways: They may comment to the family regarding how the body was handled or, in their opinion, mishandled at autopsy. And, in some situations, families may contact them for their opinion before an autopsy is performed.

In a 1992 study, 308 funeral directors and embalmers were surveyed regarding their attitudes toward autopsy. Although 80.3 percent of those surveyed believed that the autopsy served a purpose, 46.4 percent had counseled families not to allow an autopsy, and 16.6 percent did so more than half the time.

Among the commonly cited reasons that families were advised against autopsies were the funeral directors' concerns regarding potential technical problems. These included the possibility of:

- Having the arteries cut too short during autopsy, which interferes with injection and distribution of the embalming fluid
- Scalpel marks in visible areas
- A medical apparatus (such as a pacemaker) left attached to or inside the body (a still-working pacemaker could shock someone or even explode during cremation)

The above are perceived problems that rarely happen. Additional issues include delays involved with doing the autopsy, which is an issue if the family wants to have an open-casket viewing within a short time frame. A past confrontation or problem between a funeral director and someone who has performed an autopsy may turn the funeral director against autopsies in general.

The study clearly underscores the role of funeral directors in helping families make decisions on whether an autopsy should be performed and some of the biases that may influence their advice.

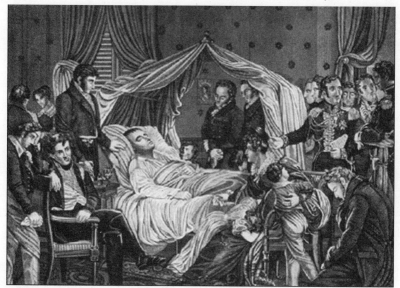

Napoleon on his deathbed.

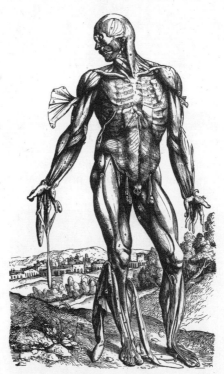

Illustration by Vesalius

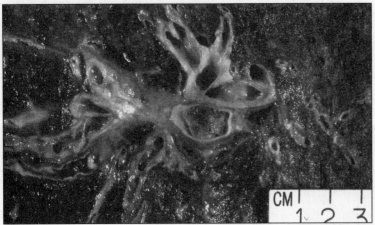

A pulmonary embolus is a blood clot that blocks an artery in the lung.

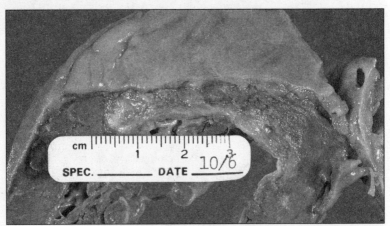

A cross section of the heart (left ventricle area), showing a white scarred region corresponding to a remote myocardial infarct (heart attack).

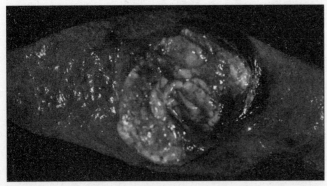

The lighter or white region of this lung represents a cancer.

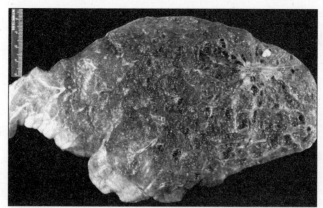

The large holes in the lungs represent emphysema caused by smoking, which has destroyed lung tissue.

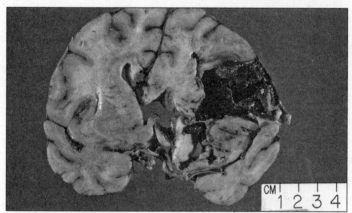

This slice of brain tissue shows a large hemorrhage.

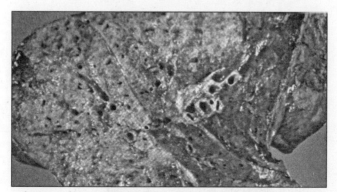

A slice of lung tissue showing pneumonia (white area) or infection in the lung's airspaces.

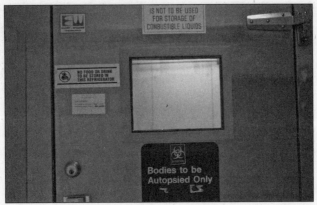

A cold-storage room is often available for storage of bodies prior to autopsy.

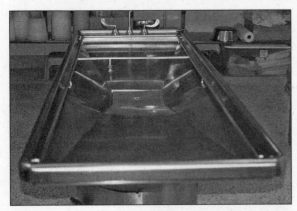

An autopsy room table upon which an autopsy is performed. The table surface is sloped toward a central drain. A water system that can spray water onto the table is present around the perimeter of the table. The height of the table is adjustable.

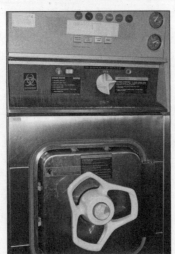

An autoclave unit is available for sterilizing equipment used during an autopsy.

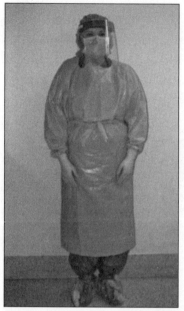

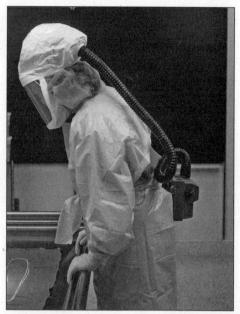

Proper protective gear including water-impermeable clothing, shoe covers, gloves, masks, and eye protection should be worn.

In certain cases, additional protection such as a special breathing mask can be used to protect the person performing the autopsy.

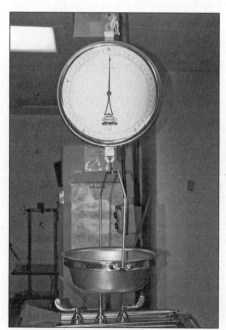

Large pan scale for measuring heavy organs, such as heart and brain. Smaller scales can be used for more accurate weight measurement of smaller organs, such as parathyroids or adrenal glands.

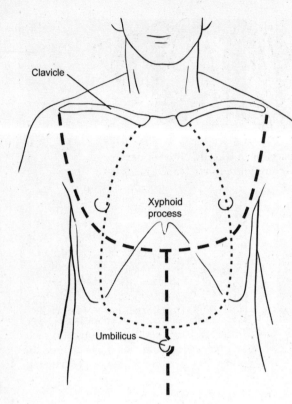

Y-shaped incision (dashes) extends across the chest (below the nipples) and downward past the umbilicus or belly button.

The skin and subcutaneous tissue are reflected back to expose the internal organs (the chest plate has already been removed in this view).

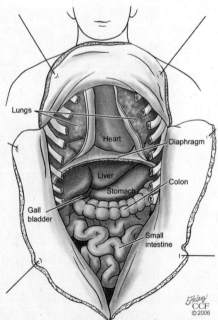

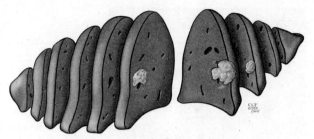

A liver that has been sectioned (sliced). Three of the cross sections reveal a focal tumorous growth (cancer).

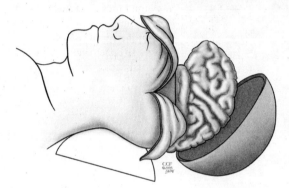

The frontal skin flap of the face is pulled down, exposing the skull. With a bone saw and hammer and chisel, the top of the skull is removed (shown here), allowing access to the brain.

Schematic drawing illustrating how the spinal cord is removed, from the posterior approach.

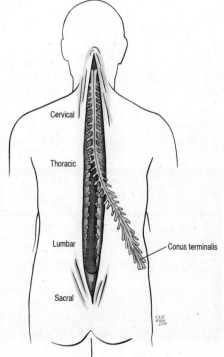

Cervical

Thoracic

Lumbar

Conus terminalis

Sacral

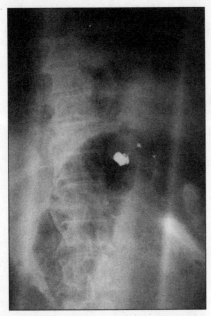

X-ray may be very useful in identifying how many bullets are in the body and exactly where they are located.

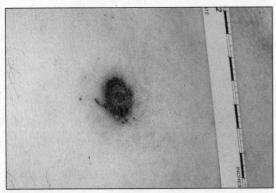

A gunshot wound is photographed for documentation. Excessive blood was wiped off before the picture was taken.

Potential evidence, such as a bullet removed at autopsy, needs to be accompanied by a proper label (as seen on the outside of the evidence envelope).

· 8 ·

WHO CONSENTS
TO AN AUTOPSY?

MICHAEL IS A 30-year-old, apparently healthy male who has terrible chest pains while shopping for groceries. Paramedics race him to the emergency room, where his chest pain subsides. He is admitted to the hospital for an evaluation, but before it is complete, Michael's heart suddenly stops. CPR is unsuccessful, and Michael dies.

What did Michael die of?

- Ventricular fibrillation (a type of cardiac rhythm disturbance or arrhythmia)?
- Myocardial infarction?
- Ruptured aortic aneurysm?
- Something else?

The physicians who cared for Michael want an autopsy to discover the cause of death.

CHAPTER 8

Michael's family arrives at the hospital and is notified of the death by a young hospital resident who has helped care for Michael. Michael's parents and wife are crying; his children hide under their mother's shawl as the resident hesitates to ask for autopsy consent. So far, he has had no real experience in making such requests, but he is clutching an informed consent document and a pen.

The resident knows the distinction between uninformed or coerced consent and informed consent, and has been trained to obtain the latter. The resident looks over the consent form, hoping that it will show him how to raise the topic of autopsy gently and pursue the process of consent. After all, the form reflects the current ethical and legal edicts by which the medical profession is monitored.

He hesitates. It does not seem prudent to go into morbid detail about the autopsy procedure, but how else can he ensure that the consent is informed?

Michael's parents are talking to his wife, already discussing the quick and proper burial of Michael's remains as their Jewish law requires. (See chapter 9 for more on religion and autopsy.) Michael's wife would like to know a definite cause of death but wonders whether an autopsy will mutilate her beloved husband's body. A wave of dread and dizziness hits her; she would like to escape the hospital and the form. Even though it is only one page long, the form seems overly detailed. How can she know what's best?

CONSIDERING CONSENT

Informed consent for autopsy is the subject of much ongoing debate, as is informed consent for medical and research procedures on living people. At the fore of the debate is the need to protect the rights of the dead person and the next of kin versus the need to use cadavers to help medical science advance.

In an ideal world, whether or not to undergo an autopsy would be decided by an informed consent model. Under normal circumstances, informed consent for medical procedures is obtained from a living patient or from the next of kin or legal guardian if the patient is incompetent or a minor. The consent form spells out the risks and benefits of the procedure so that the patient can understand what to expect from the treatment.

Consent is also required for a patient to enroll in a clinical study. In this scenario, consent is obtained after the patient is properly informed of the risks, benefits, and alternatives to whatever procedure or drug is being studied.

If consent could be obtained by an individual prior to that person's death, this would prove useful to the next of kin in deciding about autopsy. The person would have had some time to think about the decision and would have put his or her wishes in writing. Unfortunately, most people do not think about autopsy while they are still alive and therefore do not have a presigned consent form available after death that outlines their wishes.

Therapeutic risks or benefits from the results of an autopsy obviously don't affect the dead person. However, there are circumstances where findings might affect the deceased's reputation; for example, if the person were found to have acquired immune deficiency syndrome (AIDS), some people might assume that he or she was sexually promiscuous or a user of intravenous drugs.

On the other hand, there may be direct risks and benefits of an autopsy for surviving family members. Benefits include the reassurance that the deceased's treatment was well founded as well as the possibility of discovering a diagnosis that may have an impact on the living. For example, incidental autopsy findings of the specific genes BRCA1 and BRCA2, which are involved in familial breast cancer, may be the first time that family members discover their susceptibility to this type of cancer—especially when the deceased's actual cause of death was some other health problem. However, some families may not consider such a discovery a benefit, particularly if there is no known treatment for the illness discovered.

MAKING INFORMED CONSENT TRULY INFORMED

In some autopsy cases, the pathologist may need to retain organs and tissues for further examination. The organs and tissues may then be used later for medical research and education. In order for relatives to make truly informed decisions, they must know exactly how their loved one's tissues and organs will be used. *Removal* is used to determine the cause of death; *retention* indicates that body parts will be used for future research or education.

Some physicians argue that since retention is a routine autopsy practice, consent for autopsy implies consent for retention. But the fact that this practice is routine does not necessarily mean the public knows about it or believes that it is ethical to retain organs without obtaining specific permission beforehand.

Most physicians in the United States consider it necessary to mention organ retention on the consent form and to allow the next of kin to limit retention if they wish. Otherwise the consent cannot truly be called informed. The next of kin can therefore restrict the removal, retention, and disposal of some or all organs examined.

There's an interesting exception to this rule in certain states. Constitutional property rights end at death. Thus, some courts have interpreted federal and state law to exclude the necessity for consent specifically to retain organs upon obtaining consent for the autopsy, arguing that these expired "property" rights cannot be claimed by the next of kin.

In the best circumstances, the consent process can serve as a framework for a meaningful discussion between family members and the physician about the pros and cons of performing an autopsy. Truly informing a patient about the autopsy, both verbally and with a properly designed consent form, can ease apprehension and alleviate misconceptions as well as reduce the potential for future litigation. The consent is then a mutual agreement in which the agreement's implications are reasonably understood by both parties. As such, the process promotes trust in the health care system and respect for the deceased.

WHO CONSENTS: THE HIERARCHY

Laws pertaining to autopsy vary from state to state but generally require consent from the legal next of kin. The first legal next of kin is the surviving spouse. If there is no surviving spouse, consent may be obtained from (in descending order):

- An adult child
- Either parent
- An adult brother or sister
- Any other relative or person who assumes custody of the body for burial
- Anyone who is defined by written order of the deceased to serve as proxy for his or her interests

It's important to emphasize that there is a descending order of prioritization for those who can give permission for an autopsy. Not just anyone on the list above can do so. For example, if a spouse is alive, that person must be the one to sign the permit; a child's or sibling's signature would be meaningless.

INFORMATION OFTEN REQUESTED
ON AN AUTOPSY CONSENT FORM

- Name of the deceased
- Autopsy accession number (for record keeping)
- Date and time of death
- Name and signature of the individual authorizing the autopsy (the person giving consent to have the autopsy performed) and the individual's relationship to the decedent
- Date and time the authorization was given
- Description of potential restrictions to or specifications regarding the autopsy procedure
- A statement regarding tissue retention and/or disposal
- An informed consent statement
- Signature(s) of witness(es) to the signature of the consent form, including at least one individual familiar with hospital policies and local legal requirements

There are variances in the hierarchy of consent, however. In Arizona, priority is simply given to whoever assumes custody of the body for burial. South Carolina gives priority to a surviving spouse, but only if the spouse was not living apart from the decedent at the time of death. And some states specify the age of the person who may consent. In Indiana, Utah, and West Virginia, for example, 16 years is the minimum age required to give consent if all the remaining next of kin are minors.

Anyone can write an *advanced directive* to ensure that his or her wishes are followed. Most states allow an individual to consent to an autopsy in written form prior to death. In New York, a notarized card of opposition to autopsy may be carried. Nebraska, California, Nevada, and Utah allow a person to consent to or decline autopsy in a will; this directive is followed even if the will is challenged.

However, some states allow the legal next of kin to nullify predeath autopsy wishes.

The actual consent takes one of several forms. Most commonly, it is a signature on a consent form. Witnessed phone authorization or consent by telegram may also be acceptable, although the specifics of these vary between states.

SCANDALS IN THE U.K.

In recent years, several large-scale cases of British hospitals keeping body parts without consent have incited dramatic publicity. Physicians at the Alder Hey Children's Hospital in Liverpool removed and kept—without consent—the organs of 3,500 children who had died in the hospital since 1973; the bodies had been returned to their families without any indication that they were incomplete. In another case, approximately 22,000 brains and spinal cords were removed from people who died throughout England from 1970 to 1999. And, at the Bristol Royal Infirmary, the organs of more than 11,000 children who had died were retained without consent.

In response to the British cases, the U.K. Department of Health established new guidelines prioritizing consent for retention of organs and tissues as well as for their subsequent use in education and research. In addition, relatives are now to be given the opportunity to direct the ultimate disposal of any organs or tissues retained following autopsy. These guidelines have been written into law in the U.K.'s Human Tissue Act of 2004, most provisions of which became effective in April 2006.

The act goes beyond the use of decedents' tissues by requiring consent in general for *all* human samples, including those of living patients' surgical resections, biopsies, blood, urine, and sputum obtained during therapeutic and diagnostic procedures. The Tissue Act resulted from not only the country's recent spate of scandals but also the growing public interest in confidentiality issues surrounding research on tissue archives.

In fact, the Tissue Act directly addresses the issue of deoxyribonucleic acid (DNA). DNA is the most intimate of personal information. With a genotype (the unique sequence of molecular building blocks of each individual), one can identify an individual without question. In addition, we can implicate that person as being at high risk for many diseases whose occurrence and prognosis are determined at least partly by genetic contributions.

THE U.S. APPROACH

The U.S. government has debated issues similar to those in the United Kingdom, and Congress passed the Privacy Rule, which went into effect in April 2001. This rule logically follows the Health Insurance Portability and Accountability Act of 1996 (HIPAA), which prohibits health insurance companies from instituting regulations about eligibility for enrollment based on genetic information. The Privacy Rule extends privacy rights for individuals, ensuring that people find out whether and when their medical records are disclosed. Patients now must give explicit consent for each use of such data.

Autopsy consent has a nuanced position within this rule. The rule deems that privacy rights end at death; however, courts have interpreted the rule in different ways. Recognition of the family members' privacy rights must be balanced with the public interest in using autopsy-obtained tissue for research. The way in which the courts handle these laws will determine their applicability to autopsy consent in the near future.

Some people consider these acts gratuitous. After all, the argument goes, the Common Rule for the Protection of Human Subjects, enacted in 1991, already partly protects the privacy of individuals by establishing consent practices for use of tissues in research. It charges institutional review boards at each institution to ensure that confidentiality be maintained when using tissue and organs retained in archives. Autopsy tissues invariably contribute to these archives.

That rule required only a single consent from an individual for all unspecified future research. However, as with property rights, the law's language directly addresses only living patients, which we have seen may or may not extend to next of kin.

It remains to be seen whether further debate among the medical community will result in the explicit inclusion of consent for future research and education on the autopsy consent form. It seems safe to argue that, in light of privacy interests and respect for the deceased's interests, including such provisions would be the right thing to do. (For more information on ethical issues, see chapter 10).

The College of American Pathologists advocates a group of measures to promote the open dialogue between physicians and patients that is necessary to make consent informed. Institutions in the United Kingdom and the United States have already incorporated some of these methods by providing educational materials for both families and physicians, including specific alternatives to complete autopsy, such as using only needle biopsies, less invasive thoracoscopic or laparoscopic exams of the cadaver, and requiring that all organs be returned to the body.

WAIVING CONSENT

In certain circumstances, an autopsy can proceed without consent from the next of kin. These include cases of:

- Motor vehicle deaths
- Deaths of prisoners

- Patients in hospitals for the mentally ill
- Deaths associated with possible public health risks, including suspicions of contagious diseases such as tuberculosis.

Patients who die unexpectedly may be autopsied, and in some areas, patients who die within 24 hours of admission to a hospital or on the operating table may be autopsied under the jurisdiction of the coroner or medical examiner.

Consent is also waived in forensic or medicolegal cases overseen by a coroner or medical examiner. These usually involve people dying suddenly, unexpectedly, violently, in a drug-related situation, or in an otherwise suspicious way.

BACK TO MICHAEL'S WIFE

Informed consent is the best hope for families and for doctors, who daily face the delicate job of deciding what is best all around. Let's revisit the story at the beginning of this chapter. Michael's wife, like most of us, is unfamiliar with all the issues surrounding the consent form. Her interaction with the ongoing debates is limited to the form in her hand and the inexperienced physician standing before her. The form should provide her with all the information she needs to frame her choice. What does she decide?

Michael's wife gives consent for an autopsy limited to an examination of the chest region only—focused mainly on the heart and lungs. At autopsy, Michael is discovered to have myocarditis, an infection of the heart, which is ruled the cause of death.

· 9 ·

RELIGIOUS
PERSPECTIVES

AMERICANS LOOK FOR poise and peace in death. During visiting hours and at the wake, the deceased may be elegantly coiffed and dressed, surrounded by beautiful, fragrant flowers. The deceased appears to be sleeping peacefully. In fact, morticians' reputations are closely tied to how well they can make the body appear in repose. As long as the illusion of sleep remains, our fears concerning our own mortality and our concerns about facing the unknown remain in check.

But nothing disrupts this illusion more shockingly than autopsy. The idea of an autopsy—a stranger cutting open a beloved's dead body in a cold, sterile room—can be an uneasy reminder that death may *not* be a peaceful sleep.

A family that doesn't know much about the autopsy process may be apprehensive about letting doctors perform one. No matter how strong our faith may be, many of us may feel uncertain about what the afterlife holds. This is why death remains a frightening mystery for many people. So it's easy to see why some families fear the procedure. The thought of dissecting or dismembering a loved one's corpse seems almost obscene.

Some people believe that their loved one still feels pain after death and will suffer during autopsy. Others see autopsy as a terrible mutilation of the body or believe that giving permission to autopsy may keep the deceased from a union with God in the afterlife.

Although objections to autopsy may be present in some religions practiced in the United States, religion is often used as an excuse, or religious beliefs are misinterpreted, in order to avoid or circumvent the autopsy process. Here are the ways in which a few religious groups view autopsy.

THE CHRISTIAN PERSPECTIVE

Because Christianity has many denominations, it's hard to generalize Christian beliefs regarding autopsy. That said, there's no religious basis for most Christian sects (other than a few fundamentalist groups) to deny the request to autopsy for forensic, medical, and teaching purposes.

The Christian tradition of reverence for the dead springs in part from the treatment of Jesus's body, which was handled gently and lovingly after his death. The need for reverence, however, is not seen as a hindrance to autopsy by modern-day Christian leaders. For example, the Eastern Orthodox Christian Church's pastoral guidelines on the sanctity of human life, by the Reverend Dr. Stanley S. Harakas, state: "When a person dies for reasons that are uncertain, a qualified medical examiner may, with the permission of the next of kin, perform an autopsy to determine the cause of death. In some states, this is required by law. In all cases, however, the

Orthodox Church expects that the body of the deceased be treated with respect and dignity."

In the early days of Christianity, autopsies were licensed to foreign non-Christians because Christians didn't want to do them. This was common during the Middle Ages, but over time, Christian authorities began to see the value of autopsy. The devastating Black Plague of 1342–1350, for instance, spurred many autopsies of victims in an attempt to learn more about what was, at that time, a mysterious disease.

The Catholic Church approves of the practice of autopsies and allows bodies to be used for scientific research. It has even given permission for autopsies to be performed on clergymen. In fact, autopsies were requested and permitted on the bodies of many popes dating back to the 16th century, including Leo X, Adrian VI, Paul III, Paul IV, Pius V, Gregory XII, Sixtus V, and Gregory XIV. Pope Pius XII stated his approval of autopsies by saying: "The public must be educated. It must be explained with intelligence and respect that to consent explicitly or tacitly to serious damage to the integrity of the corpse, in the interest of those who are suffering, is no violation of the reverence due to the dead."

Of course, individual people and families may choose to interpret their religion in such a way as to decline an autopsy. But in general, Christianity's viewpoint is that autopsies can benefit science and the living, and therefore are completely acceptable when done with the proper respect.

THE JEWISH PERSPECTIVE

The Jewish faith has three branches: in ascending order of strictness, they are Reform, Conservative, and Orthodox Judaism. All branches demand a reverence for the body and believe that a quick burial— within 24 hours of death—is of paramount importance.

CHAPTER 9

The prevailing opinion within the Orthodox Jewish community is that autopsy is strictly forbidden. Because Judaism is greatly concerned with protecting human life, there are circumstances under which an autopsy may be performed, particularly when it might result in saving other lives. An autopsy is allowed if the procedure may reveal a genetic disease that could affect surviving relatives. Also, autopsies can be conducted to identify communicable diseases or, when mandated by law, if a capital crime has been committed. In all cases, autopsies must be limited to the specific areas where relevant information may be obtained.

It's important to show the remains dignity and respect. Here are some guidelines for conducting an autopsy according to Judaic tradition:

- Always try to expedite the release of the body as quickly as possible.
- The entire autopsy should be performed in a body pouch to retain body fluids.
- When possible, cover the entire body, and especially the genitalia, at all times.
- The autopsy procedure should be as minimal as possible. Whenever possible, avoid incision. Pathology samples should also be as small as possible. Suture all incisions tightly, and keep them as leakproof as possible.
- Upon completion, all organs should be replaced in their proper position.
- Wipe all instruments clean with a cloth, and place the cloth in the body pouch. In addition, send all blood or articles of clothing containing blood that aren't needed for pathological or evidentiary purposes along with the remains to the funeral home.
- A rabbi will be permitted to attend the autopsy upon request.

Conservative and Reform Judaism tend to interpret Jewish law in a more liberal manner than Orthodox Judaism; still, the bottom line remains that the autopsy procedure must show respect for the body.

THE ISLAMIC PERSPECTIVE

Autopsy is considered against Islamic law on the basis of a belief that the body belongs to God and should be returned to God in the best condition possible. Delay of burial, for various cultural reasons, is also a concern. However, autopsy is permitted for determining the cause of death, for other medical reasons, or if required by law. Muslim medical students are allowed to perform autopsies during their education. However, postmortems are not permitted for research or purely scientific purposes in traditional Muslim countries.

THE BUDDHIST PERSPECTIVE

If an autopsy helps to determine the cause of someone's death and that information is used to help preserve life in the future, Buddhists believe the autopsy is a compassionate act that benefits living beings. The same reasoning applies to autopsies that train medical students who will work to preserve life and health. If the autopsy is for the purpose of determining whether a death was natural or the result of murder, it is done to bring the perpetrator to justice, which is also viewed as an honorable act.

From the Buddhist standpoint, *intent* is the key word. Buddhism doesn't view autopsy as desecrating the body unless the intent of the autopsy is some kind of desecration.

A key teaching in Buddhism is that all conditioned phenomena are impermanent, which means that the physical body's natural state is one of continued aging and deterioration until death stops its functioning. Although people should care for their bodies as best they can, they should also not become overly attached to their physical forms, which will inevitably age, deteriorate, and then cease to function.

From the Buddhist standpoint, since the energy of consciousness goes on after physical death and is reborn according to one's accumulated karma, what's "left behind" is simply impermanent matter. If that remaining physical shell can be examined for the purposes of furthering education or helping to save another life, and if that examination is carried out in a way that respects the memory of the deceased, no harm is done.

Of course, there are many religions practiced in this country other than the major ones noted above. In addition, there are many people who don't follow a particular organized religion but might still object to an autopsy on the grounds of personal spiritual beliefs.

MISUNDERSTANDINGS
OF RELIGIOUS LAW

Some objections to autopsy are caused by misunderstanding the attitude of one's own religion toward the procedure.

For example, there have been cases in which Catholics adamantly objected to autopsy on the grounds that it violated their faith and burial rituals. If, for example, a brain was preserved for further testing (maybe the patient suffered from neurological disorders) and wasn't returned to the body, one might say that having the body blessed without the brain violated that religion's belief.

Despite the advice of experts on ecclesiastical law, people with such misguided interpretations of religious doctrine often cannot be swayed. Lawsuits stem from such disputes. But when legitimate objections exist, there are laws in place to ensure that such wishes will be respected. Some states, such as New York and New Jersey, have specific laws stating that autopsies cannot be performed over religious objections. However, there are exceptions for extenuating circumstances. Such situations involve public necessity, suspected criminal abuse, homicide, and the death of a prison inmate. (See chapter 8 for more on when consent is or isn't required.) Even under these circumstances, the coroner must still obtain court authorization. In the next chapter, which deals with ethical issues surrounding autopsy, we'll examine the case of Dr. X., in which religious objections are raised by a surviving husband in an effort to hide his role in his wife's death.

· 10 ·

ETHICAL ISSUES

Man is an animal with primary instincts of survival.
Consequently, his ingenuity has developed first and his soul afterwards.
Thus the progress of science is far ahead of man's ethical behavior.

—CHARLIE (SIR CHARLES SPENCER) CHAPLIN,
MY AUTOBIOGRAPHY

CHARLIE CHAPLIN WASN'T referring to autopsy, but he could have been. Because amazingly rapid developments in medicine and technology have outstripped our ability to keep up with any principles accepted communitywide concerning how to treat the dead, ethical issues have become a consideration in autopsy.

Imagine stepping out the front door of the hospital into a bright midday sun. The weather is perfect. A breeze sweeps through the parking lot as you struggle to remember where you parked. You hardly notice the daylight because in your mind you're still pacing the hallways of the intensive care unit. The constant buzz of medical staff running in and out stays in your head. You have no recollection of when you got the call about your mother. All you remember are the innumerable restless hours spent waiting with your mother and siblings, hoping that her condition would improve.

CHAPTER 10

Driving back to your house, you're in a daze.

Somehow, the fact that your mother has died hasn't sunk in.

A week later, you're in a park, holding an urn filled with your mother's ashes. In a touching ceremony with family and friends, you execute your mother's last wish to have her ashes scattered in this park, which held so many happy memories for her.

Months go by. Then you pick up the morning paper and see this headline: "Local Crematorium Dumps Bodies." Reading on, you discover that the crematory where you'd sent your mother's body has been unceremoniously dumping bodies into a mass grave and delivering to families "ashes" that were really concrete dust or made from wood chips.

How would you feel if this happened to you? In 2002, this was the case, when more than 1,000 bodies were discovered in various stages of decomposition, discarded by the Tri-State Crematory in Noble, Georgia. A national uproar accompanied the grisly discovery, and eventually more than 1,700 family members of the deceased took part in a class-action suit that was settled for tens of millions of dollars.

Another scandal alleges that body parts stolen from hundreds of corpses in New York–area funeral homes, including those belonging to *Masterpiece Theatre* host Alistair Cooke, were sold to Biomedical Tissue Services, a Fort Lee, New Jersey, tissue bank, without anyone's knowledge or consent.

In light of these gruesome cases, let's examine the ethical principles of autopsy. Most of us would agree that whether an autopsy is forensic or hospital based, it should be performed according to ethical guidelines. But what are these guidelines, and how are they decided?

Ethics, by definition, tries to identify "good and acceptable" conduct. How do we in the United States view death in the 21st century? And what ethical principles should be employed in a decision about how to handle the dead?

Several issues need to be addressed. It's beyond the scope of a book this size to discuss all the ethical ramifications in detail (some have already been touched on elsewhere in this book), but here are some of the major points that must be considered:

- Consent
- The right to privacy about the findings
- What happens to any body parts:
  - Is the body "property," and can it be handled according to the legal principles for any other kind of property?
  - Who gets to keep the parts of the body?
  - How should body parts be disposed of?
  - Can body parts be used for research or transplantation?

Our society is filled with people from different religious groups and cultures. Because of our differences, we encounter a wide array of values that enter into the decisions of what to do with, and how to treat, the dead. All groups share a fundamental respect and reverence for the human body. After all, respect for the human body after death is a way of expressing our respect for that individual's life.

It's important to keep in mind, though, that an autopsy performed to improve medical science or knowledge of diseases doesn't imply any disrespect for the deceased. Such procedures are carried out in a very respectful manner, and those who consent to them can be proud of assisting future generations of the living.

CASE STUDY: ALMOST A COVER-UP

Dr. X. was a 36-year-old Jewish physician whose husband saw her slip and hit her head on their kitchen floor. She was reportedly dazed, but remained conscious and didn't seek medical attention. Two days later, she had a seizure. A computerized tomographic (CT) scan of her head performed at a clinic revealed no abnormalities, so she went home. She subsequently experienced nausea, vomiting, headaches, and lethargy. Six days after the fall, she collapsed and become unresponsive. She was taken by ambulance to the hospital, where she was pronounced dead on arrival. During a postmortem examination, physicians noticed skin ulcers on her thighs and suspected chronic subcutaneous (under-the-skin) narcotics abuse.

Medical records revealed that Dr. X. had a history of corneal abrasions; three years ago, her physician husband had prescribed Dilaudid. She was also required to take high doses of the narcotic to help control pain following a total hip replacement, due to suppurative arthritis and osteomyelitis of the left hip. The surgery occurred one year prior to her death. At that time, her husband registered her as a habitual user of narcotics.

Due to the unknown cause of death, the interval between the fall and medical evaluation, and the suspicious nature of the physical findings, the case was referred to the medical examiner's office. After completing a purely external examination, the medical examiner noted the same characteristic skin lesions as well as recent injection sites. A postmortem skeletal series revealed a skull fracture, left hip prosthesis, and an intrauterine device (IUD).

Before the autopsy could begin, the husband was asked to identify his wife's body. He and his attorney arrived together and objected vehemently to an autopsy on religious grounds.

He denied knowing anything about the skin lesions, but when confronted with the IUD, he admitted to having frequent sexual relations with his wife. The medical examiner found it unlikely that the husband would not notice the extensive lesions, given their intimate relationship. This put the medical examiner in a difficult position.

Religious objections may be an easy excuse for someone who wants to cover up a cause of death. In the case of Dr. X., despite the threat of legal retaliation on religious grounds, the medical examiner insisted that an autopsy be performed for a number of reasons:

- The precipitating trauma was witnessed by Dr. X.'s husband alone, and the circumstances surrounding her fall were unclear.
- There was an unexplained delay between the time of Dr. X.'s fall and the time she sought medical attention.
- Her radiologist had failed to take appropriate diagnostic radiographs.
- The presence of skin ulcers and multiple injection sites raised the possibility of a suicidal, accidental, or homicidal drug overdose.

When confronted with the threat of a court order, the husband agreed reluctantly to the autopsy, despite his claims of a religious objection.

The autopsy confirmed that Dr. X. had died of craniocerebral trauma—she had slipped, hit her head, and bled into her brain. Findings of bruises on her left side and back were consistent with a backward fall, and no other injuries were noted. The pathologist also observed multiple "skin-popping scars" characteristic of chronic subcutaneous narcotism as well as needle tracks and scarring from recent injections. These telltale marks were all in different stages of healing, indicating chronic drug abuse.

Postmortem drug testing revealed the presence of a high level of the opioid analgesic meperidine (Demerol). No other drugs were found.

It came out after the autopsy that Dr. X. had a known drug problem, which her coworkers had been hesitant to reveal. Her husband, also a physician, had provided her with Demerol by writing multiple prescriptions, and this had been going on for years.

The result, instead of a neat cover-up, was that charges of professional misconduct were brought against Dr. X.'s husband. He was accused of obstructing an investigation, illegally dispensing drugs, and committing fraud in his medical practice. (He was later cleared on grounds of insufficient evidence.)

This case illustrates why some doctors are hesitant to acquiesce immediately to religious objections to autopsy. Whether this family truly objected to the procedure because of religious beliefs is unknown; however, it's clear that Dr. X.'s husband had ulterior motives. If he'd been successful at concealing his wife's drug problem by objecting to autopsy on religious grounds, he would have been able to protect himself and his family's reputation, and he could have kept his children from knowing the truth about their mother. He also would have collected insurance benefits.

CONFLICTS IN CONSENT

Who should have an autopsy, who needs an autopsy, and who should be giving permission are often complex questions. As discussed in chapter 8, one of the important decisions in hospital-based autopsies concerns who can consent to the procedure. The family's grief and the physician's interest in possibly aiding the future of medicine may set up the appearance of a conflict between the parties.

How hard should a doctor push for an autopsy, knowing that the family is grief stricken and perhaps unable to see the benefits of the procedure? What determines whether a physician has crossed the line of ethically acceptable behavior in making his request? An ethical consent certainly would not be one coerced or bullied from emotionally devastated relatives; it must be informed.

Unfortunately, pressures and outside interests can prevent an easy collaboration between families and physicians when permission to autopsy is being requested. Some conflicts lie within the medical field itself, while others rest in the innumerable values that different parts of society place on the body. Not everyone agrees on the ethics of the issues at hand: what's "good and acceptable" treatment of a body may be acceptable to one person or institution, but appalling to another.

It's not just the family that may be reluctant to autopsy. Autopsy's ability to provide quality control may not be welcomed by all physicians. Medicine deals with human life, and many patients expect that their care will be perfect. But what is perfection? Babe Ruth, baseball's legendary Sultan of Swat, had a lifetime batting average of .342, meaning that he succeeded in getting a base hit about 34 percent of the time. But what would we think of a surgeon who performed heart bypass surgery successfully only 34 percent of the time? Or even 50 percent? Standards are different in medicine, and physicians and hospitals live and die, so to speak, by their reputations.

Or what if the family actually wants an autopsy, but members of the hospital staff don't think it is necessary? They may resist because of the tremendous drain on resources that an autopsy represents to their institution. Who decides what is good and acceptable conduct under these circumstances?

It's easy to see how quickly conflict can arise. Clear guidelines will help smooth the decision-making process in difficult situations.

PROTECTING THE RIGHT TO PRIVACY

Health care is extremely sensitive to confidentiality of patient information. Many physicians believe that autopsy results should be treated with the same confidentiality that the records of a living patient receive.

Autopsy can turn up many unexpected findings. These may involve genetic information or conditions such as sexually transmitted diseases. Many people have a strong desire to leave something of themselves in the world, and this often takes the form of an image in the memory of others. If a dead person's image or reputation is tarnished by incidental findings from an autopsy, it can undercut the value of that individual's life without a chance for explanation or response.

Surviving relatives should also realize that mishandling post-mortem information could possibly hurt *them*. So any concerns about the information that might surface at an autopsy should be voiced clearly to all involved.

Many feel that information discovered at autopsy should be kept in confidence by the medical team—certainly from the public eye—and even from the deceased's own family, if that was the decedent's wish. By contrast, forensic reports are often a matter of public record and available for public scrutiny.

LEGISLATING THE USES OF BODIES

Legal issues regarding death aren't limited to health care litigation or autopsies to solve crimes. Some laws address issues of body "owner-ship" for the benefit of society, the individual, and the family. Other laws regulate the sanitary and appropriate disposal of bodies, as well as limiting and monitoring the spread of potential epidemiological agents. But the lion's share of laws surrounding a deceased person involves the protection of, and respect for, the dead individual and that person's family.

There are many potential uses for a corpse, and there are legiti-mate reasons to use one outside a medical environment, however potentially controversial these reasons might be. For instance, the government uses bodies to test new weapons—a gruesome but poten-tially life-saving endeavor if the weapons developed are designed to disable rather than kill.

On the other hand, probably no one would argue that the University of California at Los Angeles was ethical when it sold 496 cadavers, which had been donated to science and medical education, to the military for more than $700,000 over a six-year period.

Corpses also can be used for educational and artistic purposes, such as the popular "Body Worlds" exhibits, in which Dr. Gunther von Hagens had bodies dissected and their parts plasticized. These "plastinates" offer the public a unique and sometimes inspirational look at the inner workings of human bodies. However, some ethicists say that such exhibits commercialize death and are unnecessary. And the opinions on Internet blogs vary widely, showing the public's mixed emotions about displaying bodies that were once living, breathing humans.

"A corpse on display for shock value is disgusting," reads one entry.

"I thought the exhibit was fascinating," says another. "Standing next to one of the bodies was an adrenaline rush, part haunted house, part med school field trip." Such quotes sum up the exhibit's fascinating and disturbing nature.

There are also medically related uses of corpses governed by law, including the transplantation of viable organs from the bodies of the deceased into the bodies of living people. In fact, the body is potentially big business. A 2005 article in the *Boston Globe* indicated that the going rate for a whole body is $1,000 and up; quality body parts may be worth even more. However, autopsy is not some sinister way to help seedy criminals make a buck.

Use of the dead does not involve only their bodies. Decisions are needed about the body parts that are kept following autopsy, such as the tissue blocks and specimens. How long can these be retained? Is it ethical to perform research on them? When should they be disposed of, and how? These are important questions for the medical and scientific communities, as well as for the general public.

No matter how autopsy and the postmortem handling of the body are approached, the proper course of action, speaking ethically, should always return to the idea of respect. We must show respect not only for the deceased and his or her family, but also for bigger ideas, such as individual autonomy and group decision making. This includes many elements, such as respect for the wishes of the deceased individual and his or her family, for their culture and beliefs, and for the public trust.

Ethical standards may seem relative in a country as diverse as the United States, but this doesn't mean that such standards don't exist or that they should be ignored. Consideration of the human aspects of autopsy should always be the primary goal, no matter the circumstances.

COMPROMISE CAN WORK

The wishes and concerns of patients and their surviving family members must be well understood and attended to, particularly in medicolegal autopsies. If there is a conflict between the patient and the law or the medical community, an attempt at compromise should be made.

Such compromise can be reached in many different ways, such as through in-depth explanation, allowing a religious or legal representative to be present during the autopsy, performing the procedure within a reasonable period of time, or modifying the procedure itself. For example, if the next of kin requests a limited autopsy only, that request should be honored.

Finally, the public trust in medicine and the law must be upheld. Professionalism is just as much a mode of conduct as it is an image. If there's a negative perception of the medical community or medical lawmakers, open and honest communication between patients and physicians will be difficult. Well-intentioned acts and suggestions can be misinterpreted as malicious or aggressive, as society begins to rely more heavily on the law rather than on mutual understanding and respect. "Doing the right thing" then becomes the guiding force spanning the chasm between what we as a society believe should be done and what the law dictates.

For the medical community, it's unreasonable to suggest that decisions regarding autopsy could remain professional if we fulfill only the minimum requirements under the law. Do we accept minimum requirements for other laws? For instance, the U.S. Department of Agriculture sets minimum standards for food that's sold for human consumption. Among other regulations, it allows up to two maggots or ten fly eggs in every 500-gram can of tomatoes; one maggot per 250 milliliters of orange juice; and 9 milligrams of rodent droppings for every 450 grams of wheat grain. No consumer of these products would suggest that the producers try to meet only the bare minimum of USDA regulations. So too must the physician strive for standards far above those minimally dictated by the law.

It's unlikely that ethical guidelines would have stopped the gruesome events in Georgia or New York. However, they may help to make the punishment clear and prevent ethical doctors and hospitals from being associated with such heinous crimes.

Just as artists are said to reflect the current culture in their art, so must the physician reflect the changing ethics of our complex society, often before any agreed-upon ethical guidelines are available. When dealing with autopsy, we have two poles of a broad spectrum of potential actions: informed consent and the minimum requirements of the law. However, the art of true ethical action lies in the large, sometimes murky area between these two points.

As Charlie Chaplin said, the progress of science is far ahead of man's ethical behavior. Society, technology, and ethics change more rapidly than our legal infrastructure can adapt to those changes. The humanity in medical decision making is the ability to do the right thing, sometimes in the absence of clear or consistent guidelines.

We live in a colorful and complex society with diverse beliefs and views, and the only way to tailor difficult decisions to reflect our diversity is through open and honest dialogue between patient, family, and physician.

◆ II ◆

IS THE
AUTOPSY DEAD?

CURRENT PROBLEMS
FACING AUTOPSY

IN 1761, ITALIAN physician Giovanni Battista Morgagni published the first comprehensive pathology text on autopsy. *On the Seats and Causes of Diseases Investigated by Anatomy* describes in a gruesome and fascinating manner nearly 700 autopsies he performed. His work proved that illness is a physical phenomenon, not caused by humors, spirits, or other intangibles.

Morgagni's work was furthered by Sir William Osler, who in 1888 created at Johns Hopkins University School of Medicine the model for medical education that's still being used today. A key part of Osler's educational philosophy involved the use of autopsy. He had conducted more than 1,000 autopsies himself and encouraged students and staff to perform them as well. The esteemed physician and medical professor believed that students would learn more by seeing firsthand the actual causes of death in their patients than they could from memorizing textbooks.

Medical students embraced this notion, even going so far as to rob graves to obtain cadavers to practice on (since there were no body donation programs at the time).

THE RISE AND FALL OF AUTOPSY

Medical autopsy grew in popularity throughout the first half of the 20th century, and by the 1950s, nearly half of all hospital deaths were autopsied.

But since the 1950s, the autopsy rate has been declining steadily. Only 41 percent of hospital deaths were autopsied in 1964, and 34.9 percent in 1972; by 1975, the number had shrunk to 21 percent. In 1994 the autopsy rate was approximately 6 percent.

The rates of autopsy are higher at academic medical centers which are responsible for teaching medical students and residents than at nonacademic institutions, but many community hospitals do not perform autopsies at all and, in fact, discourage them.

This problem has been widely recognized in medical literature, and many inventive solutions have been proposed. *The Archives of Pathology and Laboratory Medicine,* one of the major American pathology journals, dedicated an entire issue to the problem of declining autopsy rates in 1984 and again in 1996; yet the problem persists. Currently, there's no up-to-date estimate of the autopsy rate because the federal Centers for Disease Control and Prevention's National Center for Health Statistics stopped collecting autopsy data for the national mortality database in 1994.

WHY THE DECLINE?

Why has this cornerstone of early medical education all but disappeared from modern medicine? If autopsies are such wonderful teaching tools and such crucial quality-control measures for a hospital, how can a hospital not do them?

To answer these questions, it's useful to know how the decision to perform an autopsy is made. The deceased, the next of kin, the clinician, the hospital, and the medical education establishment all play crucial roles.

After a patient dies, a specific sequence of events must take place for an autopsy to occur. Here is the typical sequence, followed by a more in-depth discussion of each step.

1. The patient's doctor has to decide that an autopsy is appropriate and should be requested. (In some instances, the family or next of kin may initiate the request for an autopsy.)
2. The doctor or someone else on the health care team must make a formal request to the legal next of kin.
3. The legal next of kin must give consent.
4. The pathologist performs the autopsy.
5. The pathologist reports the results to the clinician. The results should also be reported to the next of kin.

DECIDING TO REQUEST AN AUTOPSY

An important reason for the decline in autopsy rates is the overconfidence of physicians in modern medicine. When doctors decide not to order an autopsy, it's often because they believe that their diagnosis is correct and that an autopsy is unnecessary.

Also, physicians' improved knowledge of diseases and the incredible diagnostic tools available today allow doctors to understand a patient's disease much better than in Osler's day or during autopsy's peak in the 1950s. Many clinicians now believe there is little more that an autopsy can determine that wasn't already found when the patient was alive.

As mentioned earlier, autopsy means seeing with one's own eyes, and in the days of Osler, the autopsy was the only means to literally see the cause of death. Since then, numerous imaging technologies have been developed that let physicians see inside human bodies without using their own eyes.

Examples abound. There are X-rays and CT scans. MRIs provide three-dimensional images in great detail of soft-tissue structures such as muscles and organs. Coronary angiography allows physicians to see arterial blockages that could lead to heart attacks.

Ultrasound scans provide live, moving images of a fetus in the womb, and specialized ultrasound techniques such as echocardiography provide live images of a beating heart. Medical specialists use fiber-optic endoscopes to examine the lungs and intestinal tract directly. In addition, various tissues can be biopsied or sampled for diagnosis of a wide range of diseases.

So does all this technology make the autopsy obsolete? Are diagnoses more accurate now than they were previously? Several studies suggest otherwise.

In 1980, L. Goldman and colleagues analyzed the rate of missed diagnoses in 100 randomly selected autopsies from 1960, 1970, and 1980 at Harvard's Brigham and Women's Hospital. Despite the dramatic increase in the use of more sophisticated technologies between 1960 and 1980, including the introduction of the CT scan, ultrasound, and nuclear medicine, the rate of major missed diagnoses that would have prolonged survival, if known, was between 8 and 12 percent.

In 1988, a study compared the rates of undiagnosed conditions in both a university hospital and a community hospital. The autopsies detected unexpected findings that, had they been known to physicians, could have improved the patient survival rate by 11 percent at the university hospital and 12 percent at the community hospital.

A 2003 study determined that there had been a decrease in the rate of autopsy-detected diagnostic errors and that the rate of undetected errors was between 5 and 24 percent. This study also took into account the fact that fewer autopsies are being done and theorized that only more complex and difficult cases are being autopsied. In turn, these complex cases are more likely to uncover previously unidentified conditions.

Here's another point to consider: while doctors are often very confident that a diagnosis is correct, an autopsy always holds the possibility of revealing a mistake. Patients and their families (as well as doctors) aren't comfortable with the idea that physicians make mistakes, and it may be easier for a doctor not to order an autopsy than to risk the embarrassment of being proved wrong. Doctors may also be afraid that the revelation of an undiagnosed condition would affect their professional standing or prompt the patient's family to pursue a medical malpractice suit.

However, there's little evidence that autopsies lead to more malpractice lawsuits. In fact, autopsies have often been shown to be useful evidence in the doctor's favor when lawsuits do occur. And when doctors don't order an autopsy, it can heighten the suspicion that the doctor is trying to hide something an autopsy might turn up. Still, despite these findings, surveys reveal that clinicians' fears of malpractice lawsuits affect their decisions regarding autopsy.

Technology has greatly advanced medicine, but it hasn't prevented mistakes from being made. Sometimes it's not that imaging techniques or diagnostic tests are inadequate, but rather that the doctor may not have asked the right questions or ordered the right tests. This is a humbling reality, and the autopsy may provide an opportunity for willing clinicians to learn from their mistakes.

MAKING A FORMAL REQUEST

"Mrs. F., my name is Dr. Z. I am the attending physician in the intensive care unit. Mrs. F., your husband has died. I am very sorry; we did everything that we could.

"We would like to perform an autopsy on his body, and I would like to ask your permission to do so. This will help us ensure that that our diagnosis was correct."

Not very warm, is it? But how should a doctor ask permission to perform an autopsy?

Breaking bad news is the difficult part of being a doctor. Telling family members or friends that their loved one has died is an emotionally challenging task. And, after this news is broken, the doctor must forge ahead and ask for permission to conduct an autopsy.

The autopsy is often regarded by the public as a macabre, violent, and antiquated act. "You want to do what?" is a common response. "Hasn't he/she been through enough?" Because asking to perform an autopsy can be an awkward and uncomfortable task, many doctors just don't bother with it.

But there must be some specific way to ask for an autopsy. Aren't doctors taught how to do this? you might ask. The fact is that in many hospitals, there's no explicit protocol for how to ask for permission to autopsy, even though the concept is simple:

- State the request simply and directly.
- Explain the rationale and the potential benefits.
- Address possible concerns.

Not too tough. But few doctors ever receive any training in how to ask. Even worse, there are no rules specifying just when an autopsy should be ordered. Without clear guidelines and formal training, everything is left up to the individual clinician. Contrary to the stereotype of doctors being calm, cool, and in control of every situation, some will simply duck the opportunity to request an autopsy.

THE NEXT OF KIN MUST GIVE CONSENT

Sometimes when doctors ask for an autopsy, the next of kin refuses. One reason for this is that medicine has become deeply depersonalized. The lack of personal connection and trust between the clinician and the family of the deceased can lead to the next of kin denying permission for the autopsy. Intense stress surrounding the death of a family member can also have an impact on the surviving relatives' decision.

Often, family members aren't told the potential benefits of an autopsy. Not really knowing what an autopsy entails, families are understandably concerned about potential disfigurement or the delay of a funeral. Also, many families have religious objections to autopsy (see chapter 9). But overall, patient refusal is not a major cause of reduction in autopsy rates, as it has been demonstrated that up to 80 percent of families grant permission for an autopsy when asked.

THE PATHOLOGIST'S ROLE

So far, we've focused on the clinician's decision to ask for an autopsy and the next of kin's decision to permit one. But what about the pathologist, who actually performs the autopsy?

Some pathologists don't like doing autopsies—not because of the macabre nature of autopsy or its poor perception by the public, but because autopsies are laborious, messy, and time-consuming procedures.

Like most doctors, pathologists have many duties competing for their time. Pathologists analyze samples from living patients awaiting diagnoses, write academic papers, do research, and teach residents. Urgent analyses of a lung or liver biopsy are critical to clinical decision making and have a real impact on day-to-day patient care. An autopsy isn't generally viewed as urgent, and it certainly doesn't have an immediate effect on patient care. Autopsies generally don't lead to career advancement or academic status in pathology. And autopsy pathology is becoming a rare specialty.

This apathetic attitude among many pathologists and the low priority assigned to autopsy may lead to poorer-quality autopsies. Technicians frequently do much of the work, and autopsy quality varies widely between hospitals. As pathologists perform fewer and fewer autopsies, their experience and, subsequently, the quality of their work may not be as good as it could be.

REPORTING THE RESULTS

Clinicians have also become increasingly dissatisfied with current autopsy procedures and reports. They complain that autopsy reports are long, exceedingly technical, and not adequately focused on the clinical question of the exact cause of death. They also complain that autopsy reports take so long to arrive that the case has been all but forgotten.

ECONOMICS PLAY A LARGE PART

Another important factor in autopsy's decline is money. Pathological analyses on samples from living patients are billable to insurance companies; analyses on autopsied samples are not. Autopsy isn't billable to insurance companies. Therefore, there's a strong economic motivation for hospitals to encourage pathologists to focus on work that nets income. In many hospitals, doctors' paychecks are correlated to how much billable work they perform, so there's no incentive for an individual pathologist to perform nonbillable procedures like autopsy.

Hospitals can either bill families directly—not a particularly popular choice among grieving relatives—or absorb the cost of the procedure.

So who pays for an autopsy? The procedure requires pathologists, technicians, supplies, time, and a lab, all of which cost money. It's actually easier to answer the question, who does *not* pay for an autopsy? Private medical insurance companies definitely don't. From their standpoint, the patient is dead and no longer needs care.

It's disputed whether Medicare, the federal program that pays for health care for the elderly, pays for autopsies. Some claim that payment for autopsies is included in Medicare payments to hospitals. Part A Medicare payments cover all inpatient care. Some maintain that payment for autopsy is implicitly included in Part A payments. But there's no line-item payment for autopsy. Medicare's Part A payment to hospitals doesn't fluctuate depending on how many autopsies are performed; if a hospital performs no autopsies, that fact does not affect its Part A payments. Medicare provides no penalty for not doing autopsies and no incentive to do them.

Part B Medicare payments include all outpatient visits and typically include specific procedures in an itemized manner. Part B payments don't cover autopsy.

The financial burden of autopsies then falls on hospitals. By default, they pay for the space, supplies, and technician time. And while they don't pay pathologists to perform autopsies, they effectively lose money by having their pathologists do work that doesn't earn income for the hospital. Not surprisingly, the view of many hospital leaders is that while autopsy may be a necessary part of operations, it is an undesirable one.

FEWER—OR NO—NATIONAL STANDARDS

Many larger, systemwide pressures also contribute to the reduced rate of autopsy. National hospital accreditation organizations and those that pay for hospital services, such as health maintenance organizations, have had a profound impact on the declining rate.

The Joint Commission on the Accreditation of Healthcare Organizations sets the standards by which hospitals are accredited. Its standards help set national health care policy, and JCAHCO accreditation is essential to a facility's operation. The 1957, JCAHO bulletin indicated that "nonteaching hospitals should have at least a 20 percent autopsy rate, and teaching hospitals should have at least a 25 percent rate." This was interpreted by hospitals and physicians as a mandate.

But in 1970, the JCAHO guidelines were revised substantially to provide less specific standards and give hospitals more freedom in institutional planning so that they could adapt to a rapidly changing health care system, including the advent of HMOs. The revision included dropping all mention of autopsy rates. While autopsy rates were already in decline, the removal of this national standard set the minimum rate at 0 percent.

MEDICAL SCHOOLS MOVE AWAY FROM AUTOPSY

Autopsy has become underused as a teaching tool in medical school education. In 1905, the American Medical Association required medical students to be exposed to at least 30 autopsies, and in 1933 revised this to at least 50. But after 1944, there are no records of further requirements for autopsies in undergraduate medical education. Medical education no longer emphasizes autopsy in the curriculum, and there's significant evidence of the autopsy being underused in this arena.

The reasons have a somewhat cyclical element: (1) Fewer autopsies are being performed; hence there are fewer opportunities to include them in education. (2) Technical advances and experimental research have diminished the role of autopsy.

The impact of this is profound. Students aren't being taught that the autopsy is a valuable tool, so once these students begin practice, the idea of ordering an autopsy seems foreign. The whole culture that surrounded them throughout their education reinforced the view that autopsy isn't valuable. Once in practice, they perpetuate this complacent attitude and further it while training future physicians.

RESEARCHERS DROP AUTOPSY TOO

The autopsy is also being lost in medical research. In 1905, autopsy was one of the major ways that the cause of death was discovered and was a crucial part of medical research. If someone had a heart attack, you could find the clot that killed him; if someone had liver cancer, you could see the tumor. This gave researchers a starting point; an idea of what to study.

As the 20th century progressed, research focused more on microscopic changes. New disciplines emerged: microbiology to study bacteria and viruses, immunology to study the body's response to infection. With the recent advances in molecular biology and genetics, the study of disease has extended even beyond the microscopic to the molecular.

These changes have been coupled with astronomical gains in technology. The focus of medical research has moved away from postmortem analyses and toward experiments in the living to determine the cellular and molecular processes of disease in living patients.

CHAPTER II

STOPPING THE DECLINE

While the national rate of autopsy has been declining, a number of hospitals have bucked the trend and have maintained, or even improved, autopsy rates. Trying to find a way to improve autopsy rates at a national level, one might logically ask: how? A look at these hospitals generates some answers.

Remarkably, the importance of the autopsy appears to be built into the culture of these hospitals, thanks to influential members of the hospital administration. But these hospitals have also taken several key steps to maintain their high autopsy rate.

First, clinicians need to understand the value of autopsy. This means that the importance of autopsy needs to be infused into medical school curricula. As it's too late to alter the past medical education of current clinicians, education must be provided at the hospital to alert today's staff to the quality-control benefits of autopsy. Without the clinician's desire to have an autopsy performed, autopsy rates— and benefits—won't increase.

Then specific protocols need to be written as to how an autopsy is requested and by whom. At some hospitals, the physician pronouncing death completes a form that includes a section on autopsy and reminds physicians that such a request may be appropriate.

At other hospitals, administrative groups exist purely to facilitate all the needed actions after a patient has died. These *decedent affairs* offices ask the next of kin for the right to perform an autopsy and oversee the patient's being moved to the morgue. These offices also make sure that the body is transferred to a funeral home after the autopsy. This frees clinicians and nurses from difficult tasks and provides a specific course of action when a patient dies.

Such an approach could also facilitate communication between pathologists and clinicians and make the autopsy more of a collaborative enterprise rather than a shared burden. While such an administrative division may be expensive to operate, the costs of running it would be significantly less than many malpractice judgments against hospitals. And since autopsy results more often benefit hospitals in malpractice lawsuits, this division has the potential to pay for itself.

Pathologists could also help improve the rates of autopsy. One important step is to make sure that autopsy quality is high and consistent, and that results are reported promptly to clinicians. Autopsy reports should be written in a style that is succinct, easy to read, and clinically relevant.

The autopsy procedure could also be altered to provide more information. Instead of focusing primarily on cause of death, the procedure could be adapted to assess multiple processes including aging, immunological status, and nutrition. This information could be combined with other data, such as imaging and immunological and molecular techniques, to provide a fuller picture of the patient's condition upon death.

Updating the autopsy procedure this way could give autopsy a greater role in current medical research. This could provide us with a whole new source of important data that could be integrated into a range of research disciplines.

Making autopsy results more widely available could also bring the autopsy into research. Efforts have been made to create a national autopsy database that could be used for research projects. There's also a great need to increase the emphasis on autopsy in pathologists' training.

Systemic changes could have a significant effect in raising autopsy rates. Probably most obvious would be for the Joint Commission to reinstate a minimum requirement of autopsies in order for hospitals to be accredited.

Another simple step would be for Medicare to require a minimum autopsy payment rate. Medicare is such a crucial component of hospital finances that no hospital would risk losing Medicare funding. But hospitals would be hostile to such regulation. The cost of rapidly increasing the autopsy rate would be extremely high, and these rule changes would provide no resources for hospitals to change their practices. Such changes are likely to be unfunded mandates.

So, how could hospitals get money for autopsies? One solution is that Medicare could pay for autopsies on a case-by-case basis, by funding autopsies through Part B claims. This way, the number of autopsies performed would actually correlate to the amount of money hospitals get from Medicare. This could legitimize the requirement of a minimum autopsy rate for payment.

Another way that hospitals could get paid would be to have private insurers pay for autopsies. Assessment of health plans is dominated by two major national initiatives: the National Committee on Quality Assurance and the Health Plan Employer Data and Information Set. These initiatives examine broad measures that indicate a health plan's success, such as childhood immunization, cholesterol screening, and mammography. Large employers and providers of benefits, such as the California Public Employees' Retirement System, use these standards to evaluate which health plans to purchase for their clients.

If the pathology community could convince these initiatives that autopsy is a crucial part of quality assurance, the procedure might be added to the standards. Health insurers would then need to ensure that an adequate percentage of their patients undergo autopsy, and the best way to ensure this would be to provide funding for autopsies.

WHAT'S NEXT?

We have a health care system that has grown deeply apathetic about autopsy. Since the 1950s, the sense of autopsy's importance on all levels of health care has been lost. Clinicians do not think the procedure is worth doing, pathologists regard it as an unwanted burden, and hospitals see it as a money loser—all with the knowledge that autopsies still have great value. Numerous studies have shown that undetected diagnostic errors are still common. Hence, the autopsy as a quality-control measure is still relevant. The autopsy can be used to educate physicians about common errors in diagnosis and improve care. It also can be used in student education.

To change this situation, a number of different approaches could be taken. National policy needs to be instituted requiring minimum autopsy rates. Medical education needs to emphasize the importance of the autopsy to students and residents. Clinicians need to know how to ask for consent and how to build rapport and trust with families. Autopsies need to be carried out better and faster, and need to be integrated into medical research. And funding sources need to be established to remove the burden of payment from hospitals.

Philosophically, if we want to see the autopsy rates increase, we need to accept the concept that doctors may make mistakes. Physicians must be more humble and examine their shortcomings. Patients and families must accept the idea that their doctors are not always 100 percent correct; that missed diagnoses are a part of medicine.

Through intelligent changes in current practice and humble self-examination of its failings, medicine can continue to improve, and autopsy could play a major role in that change for the better.

REFERENCES AND ADDITIONAL SOURCES

FOR MORE INFORMATION about autopsy or other subjects discussed in this book, please refer to the sources listed below.

WEB-BASED RESOURCES

Anonymous. "Funeral." *www.absoluteastronomy.com/encyclopedia/F/FU/Funeral.htm.*

"Antony Van Leeuwenhoek." Brief biography. *www.ucmp.berkeley.edu/history/leeuwenhoek.html.*

Aristotle, complete works of. Available in full text at *http://classics.mit.edu/Aristotle*

Associated Press. "Crematory operator jailed for 12 years." *www.cnn/com/2005/LAW/01/31/cremator.case.ap/index.html* (accessed February 1, 2005).

"Babe Ruth." *www/geocities.com?colosseum/Park/1138/hof/baberuth.html.*

BBC News. "Von Hagens denies using prisoners." *http://news.bbc.co.uk/1/hi/world/europe/3420483.stm* (accessed October 27, 2005).

Collins, Simon. "Would you like rat hair with your toast sir?" (2004). *www.nzherald.co.nz/storydisplay.cfm?storyID=3588081&thesection=news&thesubbsection=general* (accessed October 27, 2005).

"Cremation." ICFA consumer resource guide. *www.icfa.org/ cremation.htm*.

"Galen" in the *International Encyclopendia of Philosophy*. *www.iep.utm .edu/g/galen.htm*.

Galen, biography. *www.hsl.virginia.edu/hs-library/historical/artifacts/ antiqua/galen.htm*.

"Gunther von Hagens." Body worlds. *www.bodyworlds.com/en/pages/ home.asp* (accessed October 27, 2005).

Jablon, Robert. "Scandal at UCLA reveals cadaver trade as big business." *www.boston.com/news/education/higher/articles/2004/03/11/ scandal_at_ ucla_reveals_cadaver_trade_as_big_business* (accessed October 27, 2005).

Laderman, G. "Silence, art and ritual." *http://seeingthedifference .berkeley.edu/laderman.htm*.

Pearson, M. "Crematorium was dump site for the dead." *http://web .lexis-nexis.com/universe/document?* (accessed October 27, 2005.)

BOOKS

Erasmus. *In Praise of Medicine*. Edited by John W. O'Malley. Toronto: University of Toronto Press, 1989.

Finkbeiner, Walter E., Richard L. Davis, and Philip Ursell. *Autopsy Pathology: A Manual and Atlas*. Philadelphia: Churchill Livingstone, 2003.

French, Roger. *William Harvey's Natural Philosophy*. Cambridge: Cambridge University Press, 1994.

Garrison, Fielding H. *An Introduction to the History of Medicine: With Medical Chronology, Suggestions for Study, and Bibliographic Data*. 4th ed. Philadelphia: W. B. Saunders Company, 1929.

O'Malley, C. D. *Andreas Vesalius of Brussels: 1514–1564.* Berkeley, CA: University of California, 1964.

Pozgar, George D. *Legal Aspects of Health Care Administration.* 9th ed. Gaithersburg, MD: Aspen Publishers, 2004.

Roach, Mary. *Stiff: The Curious Lives of Human Cadavers.* New York: W. W. Norton & Company, 2003.

Sawday, Jonathan. *The Body Emblazoned: Dissection and the Human Body in Renaissance Culture.* New York: Routledge, 1995.

Shem, Samuel. *The House of God: The Classic Novel of Life and Death in an American Hospital.* New York: Dell Publishing, 1978.

Skinner, Henry Allen. *The Origin of Medical Terms.* 3rd ed. New York: Hefner Publishing, 1970.

Spitz and Fisher's Medicolegal Investigation of Death. 3rd ed. Edited by Werner U. Spitz. Springfield, IL: Charles C. Thomas Publisher, 1993.

Wittgenstein, Ludwig. *Philosophical Investigations.* Oxford, UK: Blackwell Publishers, 1953.

ARTICLES

"Autopsy: A comprehensive review of current issues. Council on scientific affairs." *Journal of the American Medical Association* (JAMA) 258 (1987): 364–369.

Boglioli and Taff. "Religious objection to autopsy: An ethical dilemma for medical examiners." *American Journal of Forensic Medicine and Pathology* 11 (1990): 1–8.

Bove and Iery. "The role of the autopsy in medical malpractice cases, I: A review of 99 appeals court decisions." *Archives of Pathology and Laboratory Medicine* 126 (2002): 1023–1031.

Brown. "Perceptions of the autopsy: Views from the lay public and program proposals." *Human Pathology* 21 (1990): 154–158.

Chernof. "The role of managed health care organizations in autopsy reimbursement." *Archives of Pathology and Laboratory Medicine* 120 (1996): 771–772.

DeVita, Wicclair, Swanson, Valenta, and Schold. "Research involving the newly dead: An institutional response." *Critical Care Medicine: Ethical Issues in Critical Care 2003* 31: S385–S390.

Dimond. "Disposal and preparation of the body: Different religious practices." *British Journal of Nursing* 13 (2004): 547–549.

Feldman. "Rabbinic comment: Autopsy." *Mount Sinai Journal of Medicine* 51 (1984): 82–85.

Gall. "In search of the origins of modern surgical pathology." *Advances in Anatomic Pathology* 8 (2001): 1–13.

Gatrad. "Muslim customs surrounding death, bereavement, postmortem examinations, and organ transplants." *British Medical Journal* 309 (1994): 521–523.

Geller. "The autopsy in acquired immunohistochemistry syndrome: How and why." *Archives of Pathology and Laboratory Medicine* 114 (1990): 324–329.

Ghanem. "Permission for performing an autopsy: The pitfalls under Islamic law." *Medicine, Science and the Arab Law Quaterly* 4 (1989): 242–243.

Goldman, Sayson, Robbins, Cohn, Bettmann, and Weisberg. "The value of the autopsy in three medical eras." *New England Journal of Medicine* 308 (1983): 1000–1005.

Haddad. "Three famous autopsies." *Annals of Diagnostic Pathology* 3 (1999): 62–65.

Hage, Scholz, and Edwards. "Incidence and size of patent foramen ovale during the first 10 decades of life: An autopsy study of 965 normal hearts." *Mayo Clinic Proceedings* 59 (1984): 17–20.

Halperin. "Modern perspectives on halachah and medicine." *Assia-Jewish Medical Ethics* 1 (1989): 11–19.

Hanzlick. "National autopsy data dropped from the National Center for Health Statistics databases." *Journal of the American Medical Association* (JAMA) 280 (1998): 886.

Haque, Patterson, and Grafe. "High autopsy rates at a university medical center: What has gone right?" *Archives of Pathology and Laboratory Medicine* 120 (1996): 727–732.

Hasson. "Medical fallibility and the autopsy in the USA." *Journal of Evaluation of Clinical Practice* 3 (1997): 229–234.

Hasson. "The autopsy and medical fallibility: A historical perspective." *Connecticut Medicine* 65 (2001): 283–289.

Hanzlick and Baker. "Case of the month: Institutional autopsy rates." *Archives of Internal Medicine* 158 (1998): 1171–1172.

Heckerling and Williams. "Attributes of funeral directors and embalmers toward autopsy." *Archives of Pathology and Laboratory Medicine* 116 (1992): 1147–1151.

Hill and Anderson. "The recent history of the autopsy." *Archives of Pathology and Laboratory Medicine* 120 (1996): 702–712.

Hutchins and the Autopsy Committee of the College of American Pathologists. "Practice guidelines for autopsy pathology: Autopsy reporting." *Archives of Pathology and Laboratory Medicine* 119 (1995): 123–130.

Joseph, Ackerman, Talley, Johnstone, and Jupersmith. "Manifestations of coronary atherosclerosis in young trauma victims: An autopsy study." *Journal of the American College of Cardiology* 22 (1993): 459–467.

Kaufman. Autopsy. "A crucial component of human clinical investigation." *Archives of Pathology and Laboratory Medicine* 120 (1996): 767–770.

King and Meehan. "A history of the autopsy: A review." *American Journal of Pathology* 73 (1973): 514–544.

Krumbhaar. "History of the autopsy and its relation to the development of modern medicine: 'Mortui Vivos Docent.'" *Hospitals* 12 (1938): 68–71.

Landefeld, Chren, Myers, Geller, Robbins, and Goldman. "Diagnostic yield of the autopsy in a university hospital and a community hospital." *New England Journal of Medicine* 318 (1988): 1249–1254.

Landefeld and Goldman. "The autopsy in quality assurance: History, current status, and future directions." *Quality Review Bulletin: Journal of Quality Assurance* 15 (1989): 42–48.

Leikin and Watson. "Postmortem toxicology: What the dead can and cannot tell us." *Journal of Toxicology—Clinical Toxicology* 41 (2003): 47–56.

Lynn, Cobbs, and Orenstein. "Autopsy rates and diagnosis." *Journal of the American Medical Association* (JAMA) 281 (1999): 2181; author reply, 2184–2185.

Mason and Laurie. "Consent or property? Dealing with the body and its parts in the shadow of Bristol and Alder Hey." *Modern Law Review* 64 (5) (2001): 710–729.

McPhee. "Maximizing the benefits of autopsy for clinicians and families: What needs to be done." *Archives of Pathology and Laboratory Medicine* 120 (2001): 743–748.

Mittleman, Davis, Kaztl, and Graves. "Practical approach to investigative ethics and religious objections to the autopsy." *Journal of Forensic Science* 37 (1992): 824–829.

Moore, Berman, Hanzlick, Buchino, and Hutchins. "A prototype Internet autopsy data-base: 1,625 consecutive fetal and neonatal autopsy facesheets spanning 20 years." *Archives of Pathology and Laboratory Medicine* 120 (1996): 782–785.

Oppewal and Meyboom-de Jong. "Family members' experiences of autopsy." *Family Practice* 18 (2001): 304–308.

Orlowski and Vinicky. "Conflicting cultural attitudes about autopsies." *Journal of Clinical Ethics* 4 (1993): 195–197.

Park. "The criminal and the saintly body: Autopsy and dissection in Renaissance Italy." *Renaissance Quarterly* 47 (1994): 1–33.

Pellegrino. "The autopsy: Some ethical reflections on the obligations of pathologists, hospitals, families and society." *Archives of Pathology and Laboratory Medicine* 120 (1996): 739–742.

Rao and Rangwala. "Diagnostic yield from 231 autopsies in a community hospital." *American Journal of Clinical Pathology* 93 (1990): 486–490.

Riggs and Weibley. "Autopsies and the pediatric intensive care unit." *Pediatric Clinics of North America* 41 (1994): 1383–1393.

Rispler-Chaim. "The ethics of postmortem examinations in contemporary Islam." *Journal of Medical Ethics* 19 (1993): 164–168.

Rosenbaum et al. "Autopsy consent practice at U.S. teaching hospitals." *Archives of Internal Medicine* 160 (2000): 374–380.

Sarhill, LeGrand, Islambouli, Davis, and Walsh. "The terminally ill Muslim: Death and dying from Muslim perspective." *American Journal of Hospice Palliative Care* 18 (2001): 251–255.

Schmidt. "Consent for autopsies." *Journal of the American Medical Association* (JAMA) 250 (1983): 1161–1164.

Setlow. "The need for a national autopsy policy." *Archives of Pathology and Laboratory Medicine* 120 (1996): 773–777.

Shojania, Burton, McDonald, and Goldman. "Changes in rates of autopsy-detected diagnostic errors over time: A systematic review." *Journal of the American Medical Association* (JAMA) 289 (2003): 2849–2856.

Smith, Scott, and Wagner. "The necessary role of the autopsy in cardiovascular epidemiology." *Human Pathology* 29 (1998): 1469–1479.

Smith and Zumwalt. "One department's experience with increasing the autopsy rate." *Archives of Pathology and Laboratory Medicine* 108 (1984): 455–457.

Souder, Terry, and Mrak. "Autopsy 101 (CE)." *Geriatric Nursing* 24 (2003): 330–337.

Start, Dube, Cross, and Underwood. "Does funeral preference influence clinical necropsy request outcome?" *Medicine, Science and the Law* 37 (1997): 337–340.

Start, Saul, Cotton, Mathers, and Underwood. "Public perceptions of necropsy." *Journal of Clinical Pathology* 48 (1995): 497–500.

Stevanovic, Tucakovic, Dotlic, and Kanjun. "Correlation of clinical diagnoses with autopsy findings: A retrospective study of 2,145 consecutive autopsies." *Human Pathology* 17 (1986): 1225–1230.

Svendsen and Hill. "Autopsy legislation and practice in various countries." *Archives of Pathology and Laboratory Medicine* 111 (1987): 846–850.

Tedeschi. "The pathology of Bonet and Morgagni: A historical introduction to the autopsy." *Human Pathology: Perspectives in Pathology* 5 (1974): 601–603.

Vance. "Autopsies and attitudes: Where do we go from here?" *Archives of Pathology and Laboratory Medicine* 116 (1974): 1111–1112.

Virmani, Robinowitz, Geer, Breslin, Beyer, and McAllister. "Coronary artery atherosclerosis revisited in Korean War combat casualties." *Archives of Pathology and Laboratory Medicine* 111 (1987): 972–976.

Wecht. "Clinical cause of death and autopsy results." *Chest* 120 (2001): 2113–1114.

Weisz. "The papal contribution to the development of modern medicine." *Australian and New Zealand Journal of Surgery* 67 (1997): 472–475.

Wicclair. "Informed consent and research involving the newly dead." *Kennedy Institute of Ethics Journal* 12 (2002): 351–372.

Wicclair and DeVita. "Oversight of research involving the dead." *Kennedy Institute of Ethics Journal* 14 (2004): 143–164.

Womack and Jack. "Family attitudes to research using samples taken at coroner's post-mortem examinations: Review of records." *British Medical Journal* 327 (2003): 781–782.

REFERENCES AND ADDITIONAL SOURCES

TELEVISION SHOW

Mendelsohn and Cannon. "Viva Las Vegas": *CSI: Crime Scene Investigation.* CBS. Aired September 23, 2004.

OTHER

Department of Health and Family Services. Chapter HFS 136. *Embalming Standards.* November 2004, No. 587.

ACKNOWLEDGMENTS

THE AUTHORS WOULD like to acknowledge the following individuals for their help in the preparation of this book: Ms. Denise Egleton for her secretarial assistance, Ms. Beth Halasz for providing us with the medical illustrations, and Drs. Carol Farver and Philip Dvoretsky for providing photomicrographs.

NOTE ON THE AUTHORSHIP

The following contributors were medical students at the Cleveland Clinic Lerner College of Medicine of Case Western Reserve University at the time they wrote the chapters included in this book: James T. Beckmann, Seetharam C. Chadalavada, Leonid Cherkassky, Samuel T. Edwards, Carl D. Koch, Alexandra Kovach, Carl R. Peterson III, Jason O. Robertson, and Amanda L. Tencza.

INDEX

INDEX